DEVELOPING SCHOOL-BASED TOBACCO USE PREVENTION AND CESSATION PROGRAMS

Steve Sussman
Clyde W. Dent
Dee Burton
Alan W. Stacy
Brian R. Flay

SAGE Publications
International Educational and Professional Publisher
Thousand Oaks   London   New Delhi

For information address:

SAGE Publications, Inc.
2455 Teller Road
Thousand Oaks, California 91320

SAGE Publications Ltd.
6 Bonhill Street
London EC2A 4PU
United Kingdom

SAGE Publications India Pvt. Ltd.
M-32 Market
Greater Kailash I
New Delhi 110 048 India

Printed in the United States of America

Library of Congress Cataloging-in-Publication Data

Main entry under title:

Developing school-based tobacco use prevention and cessation programs
/ Steve Sussman . . . [et al.].
    p.   cm.
  Includes bibliographical references and index.
  ISBN 0-8039-4927-8.—ISBN 0-8039-4928-6 (pbk.)
    1. Teenagers—Tobacco use—United States—Prevention. 2. High
school students—Tobacco use—United States—Prevention. 3. Smoking
cessation programs—United States. I. Sussman, Steven Yale.
HV5745.D48   1995
613.85'071'273—dc20   94-33264

95 96 97 98 99   10 9 8 7 6 5 4 3 2 1

Sage Production Editor: Diane S. Foster

Contents

Foreword

Our understanding of how to prevent smoking and smokeless tobacco use in youth has evolved far since the earliest demonstrations of effective social influences programs in the late 1970s. Smoking etiology studies and prevention trials have both contributed to the evolution in prevention technology. The science of smoking prevention research has advanced along a number of fronts contributing to these advances. Measurement of smoking and its precursors has been greatly improved, and quality standards have been consensually determined. Similarly, the definition of intervention components has been greatly clarified through both experimental and theoretical contributions. Understanding has advanced, as it does in all of science, through innovation and replication. The basic contribution that has emerged from the last 20 years of tobacco use prevention research is that social influences are the major determinants of tobacco use in youth and that prevention is best served by addressing those social influences. Our understanding of which social influences are most important is coming into clearer focus, and this, together with how to most effectively address those influences, is the dominant concern in tobacco prevention research today. We began this journey in the middle 1970s primarily from a position of faith, faith that the findings and methods developed and refined largely in American social psychology laboratories could be applied to the public health problem of cigarette smoking. Our faith in the firmness of the scientific ground from which we launched our journey would appear to have been justified even if our understanding of what we were undertaking was naive. Tobacco use prevention research has taken on a theoretical and methodological life of its own, incorporating elements of cognitive, behavioral, sociological, social systems, community organization, epidemiological, public policy, and even pharmacological research. Advancements in tobacco use prevention research have contributed in important ways to other public health and social research as well, including public health nutrition studies, HIV and other sexually transmitted disease research, teenage pregnancy prevention, accident prevention, and, most directly and demonstrably, alcohol and other drug abuse prevention. Research on smoking cessation in youth has been less common and has not advanced as far.

This book is in the best tradition of tobacco use prevention research. It reports the contributions of a major program of research in tobacco use etiology and prevention; further, by attending to details that typically go unreported in research papers, it contributes to our understanding of the processes of social influences in tobacco use and presents methodological advancements that set new standards and provide new opportunities for prevention research.

This book makes a number of important contributions, including identification of sets of strategies useful for tobacco use prevention and cessation. It draws attention to the special concerns of smokeless tobacco use, its precursors, and promising strategies for prevention and cessation. The authors provide an empirically based admonition not to forsake health education in the traditional sense (with consideration for the health consequences of tobacco use). Many researchers and program developers will find useful the guidelines and examples of how to do good formative research leading up to program production, and clear and detailed descriptions of how to carry out high-quality process and outcome evaluation in a complex program of tobacco use prevention and cessation research. The description of a methodology for efficiently obtaining active informed consent in a large population study is particularly useful to the researcher caught between the desire to do research of the highest scientific standards and prevailing ethical and societal constraints.

The prevention research developed here makes a distinction between normative and informational interventions. Normative interventions, a way of intervening operationalized by Sussman, Dent, Stacy, Hodgson, et al. (1993), are not to be confused with normative influences. Experimental epidemiological findings (MacKinnon et al., 1991; Johnson et al., 1990) and trials designed to test directly the impact of interventions on normative beliefs (Hansen & Graham, 1991) both indicate that modified normative beliefs, specifically the perceived prevalence of use by friends and anticipated social consequences of use (acceptance or rejection by friends) are among the most effective mediators of prevention program effectiveness. The distinction made by Sussman, Dent, Stacy, Hodgson, et al. (1993) is whether it is more effective to intervene on norms (and other potential outcome mediators) primarily through an informational strategy or through alternative norms modification strategies. The results of the prevention trial are not, therefore, inconsistent with those reported previously by others, but suggest that perceptions of norms, skills, and other social variables and intervention strategies to alter those perceptions and subsequent tobacco use behavior should be viewed orthogonally with an eye toward what works best to palliate the social influences to use tobacco. As they stand, the interventions are complex, and lines of demarcation between the information and normative programs are multiple. This research should stimulate further discussion and research on strategies for modifying tobacco use and its precursors. Hopefully, it will encourage future clarification of critical influence variables and their definitions.

The finding that a physiological education intervention was effective in reducing tobacco use is intriguing. Whether that finding is attributable to increased concern for and efficacy regarding health consequences or to higher levels of student interest and involvement and health educator enthusiasm is, as observed, difficult to tease out. Indeed, it is hard to achieve equivalent levels of enthusiasm and involvement in a multicomponent trial. Undoubtedly investigators will attempt to replicate these findings, controlling for potential confounds. If the findings hold up under the scrutiny of scientific replication, they will go a long way towards rehabilitating "physical consequences" as a productive avenue to tobacco use prevention.

The cessation research described in this volume is similarly imaginative and methodical. By their ingenuity and attention to detail, the investigators have accomplished what many have had difficulty in achieving, a successful school-based cessation intervention, and have demonstrated the value of focusing on social as well as affective influences on smoking in adolescent cessation programs.

In this time of escalating health care costs—up from 7% of the GNP of 17 years ago, when research on social influences in prevention began, to more than 14% now—it is essential that we pay more attention to prevention. Of course, the final rationale is that we must prevent disease and suffering when we can, not how much prevention costs relative to treatment. Chronic tobacco use, which accounts for 25% of premature mortality and untold suffering in this country, is preventable. Our knowledge of how to prevent tobacco use and bring about early cessation is considerably advanced by this volume. The meticulous detail in which program development and evaluation are described here should be useful both to researchers and health educators alike.

C. Anderson Johnson, Ph.D.
Sidney R. Garfield Chair in Health Sciences
Director, Institute for Health Promotion and
Disease Prevention Research
University of Southern California

Preface

My colleagues and I wrote this book in order to provide a health researcher's perspective regarding the history, status, and needs within school-based tobacco use prevention and cessation research. Summaries of etiological theories are available; meta-analyses of studies exist; even consensus statements regarding the content of successful programs exist. None of these sources, however, provides information on how to develop and implement a research program. None of these sources speaks candidly of some of the practical difficulties involved in engaging in this research and implementing such programs in practice. None of these sources has tried to pull together all of the different issues in one place. This text accomplishes these tasks and also makes recommendations regarding new studies needed to help provide more informative research paths that take into account remaining needs in such areas as basic research and diffusion research.

This source also contains some unique substantive material. There are few books in the field that deal with school-based tobacco use prevention *and* cessation together. Also, very little research exists regarding smokeless tobacco education for youth, a topic about which the book will present much information. This book is the result of over 15 years of work on the part of our research team. It summarizes the work of fellow investigators, health educators, data collectors, data analysts, and administrators, and is constructed around a project we recently completed.

The book begins by providing a brief overview of the history of school-based tobacco use prevention and cessation programs. There are several program options, several competing theoretical perspectives, and several methodological approaches to consider. We then describe the development and implementation of Project Towards No Tobacco Use (Project TNT), a 5-year grant funded by the National Cancer Institute (NCI). In describing Project TNT, this book will (a) present the major theoretical and methodological issues involved in the development of such programs, and (b) help researchers and practitioners in their efforts to develop or select good programs. For example, we describe issues concerning curriculum development, different methods of developing curricula, and curricula content material. Also, we describe issues of subject selection, assignment, tracking and attrition, analysis, and other methodological and statistical considerations. Finally, we discuss applicability of these methods and curricula products to other research areas and make suggestions for future research.

The primary market for this book includes researchers and practitioners in public health education, especially those involved in adolescent tobacco research or practice. Graduate students involved in the field of disease prevention and health promotion may find this book relevant to their studies. Policy makers and those involved in program development also may be interested to some degree.

I owe much to colleagues that helped me take a leading role in this effort. Brian Flay introduced me to the field of school-based research. He provided me with the opportunity to vigorously pursue research in this area, and I am very glad that he serves as coauthor of this book. I also owe thanks to the other coauthors. Clyde Dent served as the Project TNT statistician. He served as co-principal investigator on Project TNT, and he has had over 10 years' experience in the tobacco use prevention and cessation field, including the areas of biochemical validation of tobacco use and school-based research. Dee Burton served as the Project TNT cessation expert. She has contributed extensively to smoking cessation efforts among adults and children, and she created this component of the project. Alan Stacy served as the Project TNT generalist, helping on theoretical issues or on methodological ones when needed. He is a leading authority on outcome expectancy research and memory ties to tobacco use development. Bill Hansen, though not a coauthor on this book, served as a co-investigator on Project TNT. He taught me how a large research project can be successfully run, and he provided a variety of ideas though his own work in this area.

Sande Craig served as the project manager on Project TNT. She was responsible for coordinating all project personnel activities, maintaining school contacts, and managing field coordination tasks. She minimized individual difference variables among health educators that could interfere with the interpretation of the results, and she was responsible for ensuring equivalence of program delivery. She made the project work.

Marny Barovich, Ginger Hahn, Ann Raynor, and Eva Klein-Selski served as the primary developers of the Project TNT prevention curricula, under the supervision of Sande Craig and myself. Not only did they do an excellent job in writing and delivery aspects of health education, they also are coauthors on several project research papers.

Amy Custer-Smith served as the primary data coordinator. She has served as school data collection coordinator for several institute projects, and she has considerable expertise in coordination of data collection activities, including student tracking procedures. She was responsible for ensuring high participation of students during all points in data collection, as well as overseeing data collection, editing, and coding and entry tasks, and scheduling hourly staff. She was assisted by Antoinette Carrillo, Leticia Vasquez, Sarah Gildea, and Jody McCord, as well as by a great team of data collectors. I also thank all of the participating district and school personnel for their interest and enthusiasm in helping us to complete our shared goals.

I would like to thank Linda Johnson and Jolanda Lisath for their support as project secretaries. Further, I thank Jolanda Lisath for her patience and assistance in helping to prepare the manuscript, Beth Howard for editorial assistance on an early draft of the book, and Christine Smedley, our editor, and two anonymous reviewers for numerous editorial comments.

Ventura Charlin, Jon Galaif, and Ping Sun served as data specialists for this project. They edited codebooks, helped develop data coding schemes, were responsible for all data management, including maintaining the student tracking database, and assisted in data entry and data analysis.

There are several other people my coauthors and I want to thank. Our project officers at NCI, Gayle Boyd, Tom Glynn, Sherry Mills, and Craig Stotts, provided us with great support during the course of our grant. They pushed for integrative work, which helped lead to some of the information here. Richard Evans, Tom DiLorenzo, Carol D'Onofrio, John Elder, Herbert Severson, Arthur Peterson, Vic Stevens, Steven Schinke, and their colleagues provided us with their expertise as principal investigators of NCI-funded smokeless tobacco prevention and cessation research. Larry Seitz, our project officer at the National Institute on Drug Abuse, permitted us to extend the scope of our efforts in curriculum development, which contributed to the enrichment of this book. The faculty of the Institute for Health Promotion and Disease Prevention, including John Graham, Gary Marks, Mary Ann Pentz, Jim Dwyer, and Jean Richardson, provided valuable input into the scientific development of this project. Finally, we would like to thank C. Anderson Johnson, Ph.D., Sidney R. Garfield Chair in Health Sciences and Director of the Institute for Health Promotion and Disease Prevention, for providing us with the research environment that allowed this study to happen.

PART ONE

Foundations of School-Based Adolescent Tobacco Use Prevention and Cessation Programs

Part One provides the foundation for the work that follows. The problem is introduced in Chapter 1, which provides an overview of tobacco use prevalence and associated health risks. In Chapter 2, the general focus and content of school-based prevention and cessation programs are discussed, including the costs and benefits of prevention versus cessation programming, the perspective of the authors on school-based tobacco use prevention and cessation research, and an introduction to social-influences-oriented programming. Chapter 3 concludes with a discussion on the history of school-based tobacco use prevention research. Information on the history of tobacco use cessation research is provided in Part Four (Chapter 10), where a more comprehensive discussion of adolescent cessation issues is provided.

ONE

Beginnings: Tobacco Use Prevalence and Consequences

DEFINITIONS OF TOBACCO PRODUCTS

Although most adults are aware that tobacco use can involve many different types of products, many adolescents have only a partial understanding of tobacco's many forms and uses. The following text has been used successfully in the research to define and describe tobacco products for a 7th-grade population:

CIGARETTES are made from a light-colored tobacco which is rolled in paper and smoked. Users may roll their own cigarettes, using tobacco sold in a pouch and precut papers, or they may purchase finished cigarettes in such commercial brands as Marlboro, Winston, Camel, or Kools.

CLOVE CIGARETTES are made with cloves as well as tobacco but contain more tobacco than cloves. They are more expensive than cigarettes.

CIGARS are made from a darker tobacco wrapped in tobacco leaves. They are brown in color.

PIPE tobacco usually is mixed with other materials and is smoked in a pipe. People usually do not inhale cigar or pipe tobacco.

SMOKELESS TOBACCO (also called "spit" tobacco) consists of all tobacco-containing products which are not smoked. It is made from dark leaves and comes in two main forms—snuff and chewing tobacco.

SNUFF is finely cut or powdered tobacco. There is a dry powdered form such as Levi Garrett, and a slightly damp form called "moist snuff," such as Skoal or Copenhagen.

CHEWING TOBACCO is made from large pieces of a tobacco leaf that comes in three forms: (1) loose leaf comes in pouches, such as Red Man, Mail Pouch, or Beechnut; (2) plug comes in plastic wrapped bars, such as Day's Work; and (3) twist-and-roll is twisted into a pig-tail shape and comes in a wrapper, such as Mammoth Cave. (Hahn et al., 1989, p. 27)

TOBACCO USE PREVALENCE

Tobacco use prevalence is generally defined in terms of one or more measures of behavior: (a) ever tried; (b) some measure of cumulative use; or (c) regular use. A primary measure of regular use is weekly use behavior—use of tobacco, on the average, at least once a week or with greater frequency.

Data collected in this research arena indicate that young adolescence is the age at which most young people begin to experiment with tobacco products. For example, among southern California youth who have not participated in effective tobacco use prevention programs, 60% of 7th-grade students, 65% of 8th-grade students, and 70% of 9th-grade students have tried smoking. Cumulative lifetime use of 20 or more times is reported by 6% of 7th-grade students, 9% of 8th-grade students, and 12% of 9th-grade students. Weekly smoking prevalence jumps from 2% to between 4.5% and 6% in 7th grade, and continues to rise 3% per year throughout high school (e.g., U.S. Department of Health and Human Services [U.S. DHHS], 1989, chap. 5). Similar rates have been observed in other parts of the country (Bauman, Koch, Fisher, & Bryan, 1989).

Sales of smokeless tobacco products have increased an average of 11% over the past 20 years overall, but only 4% to persons over

18 years of age. Thus although a high percentage of the current 7 to 22 million smokeless tobacco users are adults, an increasing number of teenagers are also using these products (Boyd & Associates, 1987). In suburban/rural California, 56% of 7th and 8th-grade males report having tried smokeless tobacco, approximately 26% report a cumulative lifetime use of between 2 and 20 times and 14% report a cumulative lifetime use of greater than 20 times. Among urban/suburban southern California 7th-grade males, 25% to 30% report having tried smokeless tobacco, approximately 10% report a cumulative lifetime use of between 2 and 20 times, and 4% report a cumulative use of 20 or more times. Weekly smokeless tobacco use is 2% in the 7th grade (5% or more among white males), increasing at 1% to 3% per year. Smokeless tobacco use prevalence is somewhat lower in the Northeast than in the West, slightly higher in the Midwest, and considerably higher in the South (Braverman, D'Onofrio, & Moskowitz, 1989; Marcus, Crane, Shopland, & Lynn, 1989; Novotny, Pierce, Fiore, & Davis, 1989; Rouse, 1989). These figures seem to point to the need to provide tobacco education to our nation's youth by the time they reach early adolescence, before habits and addictions become established.

Gender Differences

Although males and females are very similar in their levels of cigarette use, they differ considerably in their use of smokeless tobacco products in that far more males than females use smokeless tobacco. Figures 1.1 to 1.4 demonstrate the different patterns of use for males and females among the Project TNT schools (approximate $N = 7,000$).

Ethnic Differences

Tobacco use prevalence also differs among various ethnic groups. Figures 1.5 and 1.6 illustrate comparisons between Latino and white, non-Latino students. Although weekly use of cigarettes is similar for young adolescents in both ethnic groups, the prevalence

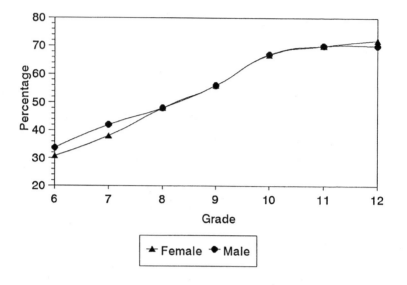

Figure 1.1. Trial of Cigarette Smoking, by Gender

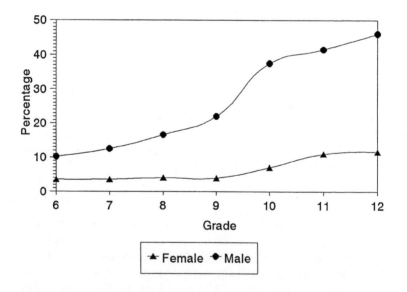

Figure 1.2. Trial of Smokeless Tobacco Use, by Gender

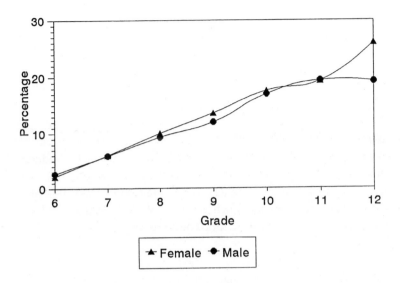

Figure 1.3. Weekly Cigarette Smoking, by Gender

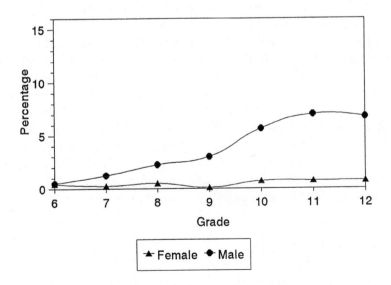

Figure 1.4. Weekly Smokeless Tobacco Use, by Gender

of use among white, non-Latino smokers increases more over time than for Latino students. Because smokeless tobacco is used far more by males than by females, the prevalence of smokeless tobacco use by white non-Latino students and Latino students was compared in Figures 1.7 and 1.8 for male students only. White non-Latino male students report a higher prevalence rate of smokeless tobacco use than Latino male students. It must be noted that across all 48 junior high schools in Project TNT, only 7% of the sample was composed of African American students and only 6% was composed of Asian or Native American students (see Chapter 9). Thus a graphical depiction of their use would not be accurate. These groups showed slightly lower use of cigarettes and much lower use of smokeless tobacco than their Latino and white non-Latino counterparts.

Regional Differences

Although at least two studies suggest that the incidence of cigarette smoking is no higher in rural than in urban regions (Alexander & Klassen, 1988; Sarvela & McClendon, 1987), most studies indicate that the incidence of smokeless tobacco use is higher in rural than in urban areas (Boyd & Associates, 1987). Data gathered in this study, however, indicate that among southern California adolescents, the prevalence of cigarette smoking and smokeless tobacco use is somewhat higher in rural than in urban regions. From our project, for example, 50% of all students in rural areas have tried cigarettes by 8th grade, compared with 44% in urban regions. Likewise, weekly smoking in 8th grade was 11% for the rural schools and 8% for urban schools. Trial use of smokeless tobacco by 8th grade was 11% in rural areas and 8% in urban areas. The prevalence rate for weekly use of smokeless tobacco in 8th grade was 2% for the rural schools and 1% for urban schools.

Brands Used in California

Hahn et al. (1990) investigated cigarette and smokeless tobacco experimentation using structured, open-ended interviews. In the

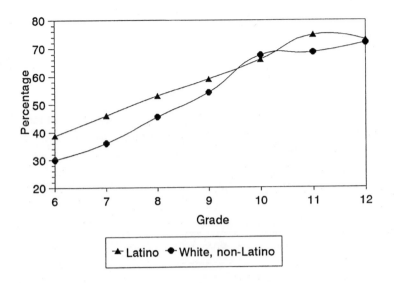

Figure 1.5. Trial of Cigarette Smoking, by Ethnic Group

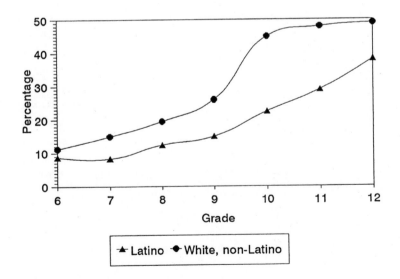

Figure 1.6. Trial of Smokeless Tobacco Use for Males, by Ethnic Group

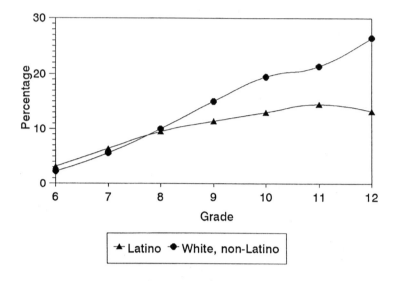

Figure 1.7. Weekly Cigarette Smoking, by Ethnic Group

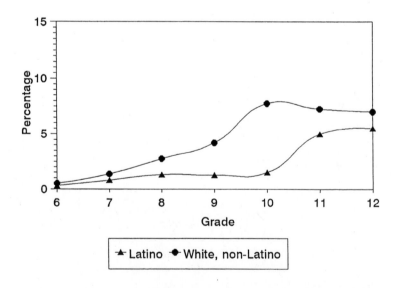

Figure 1.8. Weekly Smokeless Tobacco Use for Males, by Ethnic Group

fall of 1987, data were collected from a sample of 320 southern California 7th- and 10th-grade students. The cigarette brand of choice for both first experimentation and most recent use among 61% of these students was Marlboro. Johnson, Dent, Sussman, and Sanford (1993) have noted, however, that Camel cigarettes are becoming increasingly popular. Statewide data collected in 1990 indicated that Marlboro was used by 42% of the teenagers surveyed, and Camel was used by 29% (Pierce et al., 1991). The proportion of smokers under 18 years old who prefer Camel cigarettes over other brands rose from 0.5% to 33% in 4 years (U.S. DHHS, 1994, p. 191). Camel's apparent rise in popularity among adolescents may be due, at least in part, to the use of the "Joe Camel" advertising campaign. Although purported to be targeted exclusively toward adults, this campaign uses cartoon-like images centered on apparent themes of sex and rebellion.

The brand of choice in the Hahn et al. (1990) study regarding first trial of smokeless tobacco was Skoal (51%), with Copenhagen being a second choice (15%). In an examination of the brand used most recently by students, Skoal remained the first choice with 39.7% of the students, but 22.6% reported using Copenhagen. Skoal has a relatively high nicotine level (10.7 mg/g), but Copenhagen's is even higher (20.7 mg/g) (Severson, 1992). The apparent trend for the percentage of subjects using Skoal to decrease, and the percentage using Copenhagen to increase, seems to suggest that students switched to the higher-nicotine-level product over time. It was also noted that subjects did not use a low-nicotine-content brand (such as Skoal Bandits) for trial use of smokeless tobacco. These data on most popular brands of cigarettes and smokeless tobacco are consistent with data collected in other states (Ernster, 1989; Johnson et al., 1993).

HEALTH CONSEQUENCES OF SMOKING AND SMOKELESS TOBACCO USE

The Project TNT Curricula summarizes the consequences of tobacco use (at a 7th-grade reading level) as follows:

The dangerous components of cigarettes, clove cigarettes, cigars and pipe tobacco include tar and carbon monoxide gas, which are given off when burned. Nicotine, the substance you get addicted to, is in all forms of tobacco. It makes the person's body work faster, which can cause heart disease. Cigarettes, smokeless tobacco, cigars, and pipes also have huge amounts of cancer-causing materials in them which cause cancer at places where tobacco touches the body. (Hahn et al., 1989, p. 27)

The consequences of tobacco use are now well known (e.g., U.S. DHHS, 1984, 1985, 1988, 1990, 1991a, 1991b). The overall mortality rate for cigarette smokers as compared to nonsmokers is about 1.7, or nearly twice as high. Cigarette smoking is the leading behavioral cause of lung cancer, other respiratory diseases, and heart disease—and of the deaths resulting from those diseases. Moreover, the mortality rate for all cancers combined is about twice as high in smokers as in nonsmokers. Approximately 85% of lung cancer mortality and 33% of mortality from other cancers may be attributed to cigarette smoking. The 5-year survival rate for lung cancer is 10%, and has not improved in 15 years. Cigarette smoking is also a leading risk factor for cancers of the larynx, oral cavity, esophagus, urinary bladder, and pancreas, among others.

The mortality rate of all cardiovascular diseases combined is about 1.5 times higher in smokers than in nonsmokers. Cigarette smokers are 75% more likely to die of coronary heart disease than nonsmokers, 25% more likely to die of cerebral lesions, 300% more likely to die of aortic aneurysms, and twice as likely to die from the consequences of arteriosclerosis. Infants born to mothers who smoke have an increased risk of perinatal mortality and low infant birth weight, and may experience inhibited development for the first several years of their lives.

Tobacco smoke contains more than 40 known carcinogens. These are carried via sidestream smoke into the surrounding air, where they can affect smokers and nonsmokers alike. Sidestream smoke actually contains higher concentrations of toxic and carcinogenic chemicals than the mainstream smoke inhaled by smokers. The ingestion of "secondhand" smoke, also referred to as "passive smoking," can result in serious health consequences. Passive exposure to cigarette smoke has been linked to respiratory disorders in children and to lung cancer (e.g., Fielding & Phenow, 1988; Repace & Lowrey, 1987). Passive smoking in infants can result in elevated risks for birth defects, low birth weight, and preterm births (relative risk = 1.2), and alimentary and respiratory illnesses (e.g., Greenberg et al., 1991; Jones, Schiffman, Kurman, Jacob, & Benowitz, 1991). Women exposed to passive smoke are at elevated risk for breast cancer, lung cancer (relative risk = 1.32 to 2.2; ≤19 cigarettes per day, relative risk = 1.16; ≥20 cigarettes per day, relative risk = 3.35 in some studies), arteriosclerotic heart disease (relative risk = 1.24; relative risk for men exposed to smoke = 1.31), and other cancers (relative risk = 1.16). Prolonged lifetime exposure may also contribute to the development of chronic obstructive pulmonary disease.

Ten to 15% of all people with allergies are allergic to tobacco smoke, resulting in skin or mucous membrane reactions or asthmatic attacks (Schmidt, 1986). Passive smoking may also be an important cause of bronchitis and pneumonia, and children of smokers report a higher incidence of airway inflammation than children of nonsmokers (see U.S. DHHS, 1993).

At least 300 studies identify the numerous side effects of smokeless tobacco use. These include nicotine addiction, adverse effects on fetal outcomes and placental morphology, suppressed immunologic response, discolored teeth, decreased capacity to taste and smell, gum recession, and destruction of soft and hard oral tissues (Connolly et al., 1986; Kenton & Blot, 1986; U.S. DHHS, 1986). Further studies indicate that long-term use could result in high blood pressure and oral cancer. Approximately 40% of daily users (those who use roughly five dips or chews per day) may develop oral lesions after 3½ years of use, with the malignancy transformation rate for these lesions reported to be about 4%. This means that approximately 1.5% of regular users of smokeless tobacco may develop oral cancer, which often requires surgery to remove portions of the mouth and may result in death. On February 3, 1986, the U.S. House of Representatives passed legislation banning all radio and television advertising of smokeless tobacco and requiring that health warning labels be placed on all smokeless tobacco packages, alerting the public to the dangers of oral cancer and gum disease associated with its use. Former Surgeon General C. E. Koop made an announcement on February 25, 1986 (and subsequently released a written report), declaring the use of snuff and chewing tobacco products to be a significant health risk that can lead to addiction and cancer.

PREVALENCE AND HEALTH CONSEQUENCES OF CIGAR AND PIPE SMOKING

Currently, approximately 8% of adult males smoke cigars and 5% smoke pipes. Although the use of these products has declined 80% since 1964, their use remains a significant health problem. Heavy pipe and cigar smoking (five or more pipefuls or cigars a day), particularly if inhaled, results in risks as significant as those reported for cigarette smoking. Contact with smoke from cigars and pipes increases the risk of cancer of the mouth, pharynx, esophagus, larynx, and lung. Cigarette smokers who switch to cigars or pipes generally continue to smoke as before, resulting in no risk reduction. Those who smoke five or more cigars or pipefuls per day are 3 to 6 times more likely, and those who inhale are 12 times more likely, to contract lung cancer than nonusers (e.g., Higgins, Mahan, & Wynder, 1988).

Focus and Content of Prevention and Cessation Programs

Chapter 2 presents the conceptual distinctions between prevention and cessation as adolescent tobacco use interventions. Alternative program options in schools, and the focus of current tobacco
use prevention and cessation curricula, are also discussed.

ARGUMENTS IN FAVOR OF ADOLESCENT PREVENTION OR CESSATION PROGRAMMING

Prevention and cessation are two approaches toward controlling the occurrence of a behavior or event: Prevention attempts to
stop a future behavior, and cessation attempts to stop a present
behavior. Primary prevention of tobacco use involves prevention
of early experimentation, whereas secondary prevention deals
with prevention of higher levels of use or disease. Tertiary prevention deals with prevention of worsening of a disease or death. The
approach of cessation is to stop a behavior so that the person can
recover physically and psychologically.

The choice between a prevention and a cessation approach is
not always clear. For example, a teenager may have been smoking
a few times a week for the past 4 months. This teenager is not
strongly addicted to tobacco. The prevention stance would argue

that this teenager should be prevented from continued use that might lead to addiction. The cessation stance would argue that this teenager should stop use now so that he or she will stop suffering the current consequences of tobacco use, which could include coughing or the beginnings of addiction. Which approach will be most successful for health promotion efforts (i.e., getting the highest number of teenagers to not use tobacco)—one that emphasizes changing the course of future events, or one that emphasizes recovering from the present situation?

Several factors have led to the suggestion that prevention may be more efficacious than cessation among adolescents:

1. There are high relapse rates in adult cessation programs; perhaps prevention might halt the addiction process that makes cessation so difficult.
2. Some physical damage or "locking into" a course of addiction could already have occurred among youth in adolescent cessation programs; earlier education may prevent such damage.
3. Prevention programs can reach wide audiences through involvement with school systems.
4. The dynamic nature of tobacco use among adolescents makes it difficult to identify appropriate targets of cessation efforts (Pallonen, Murray, Schmid, Pirie, & Luepker, 1990).
5. It may be difficult to recruit adolescents into cessation programs.
6. As a policy, a prevention stance may be more successful at keeping tobacco use levels at a school low. A cessation stance could lead to higher levels of tobacco use because youth are not "ready" to quit (Pentz, Brannon, et al., 1989).
7. It may be difficult to decrease use among teenagers once they use regularly because the danger of health consequences may seem remote and only likely to present itself in the distant future. Because teenagers seem to be more highly motivated by circumstances occurring in the "here and now," they may be unlikely candidates for participation in cessation programming.

Other factors support the need for adolescent cessation research:

1. Youth at highest risk may not benefit by prevention programming. They may only benefit when they perceive some costs occurring to them making them appropriate candidates for early cessation efforts.

2. Little research has been completed regarding adolescent cessation; some empirical investigation of its feasibility would be helpful. Perhaps the strongest argument for adolescent cessation programming is the paucity of data about its feasibility. One can conjecture that it will or will not work, but this is an empirical question. At present, few attempts have been made to study the maintenance of smokeless tobacco and cigarette use among teenagers (Chassin et al., 1984; Chassin, Presson, Sherman, McLaughlin, & Goila, 1985; Hansen, Collins, Johnson, & Graham, 1985; Skinner, Massey, Krohn, & Lauer, 1985) and to provide cessation programming (Lotecka & MacWhinney, 1983). Maintenance variables for cigarette smoking include having relatively positive beliefs about smoking, having higher self-reported rebelliousness, and being more likely to have friends and parents who have smoked (Chassin et al., 1984; Hansen, Collins, Johnson, & Graham, 1985; Skinner et al., 1985). Successful smoking cessation programming may be associated with manipulation of these maintenance variables through decision-making and coping skills strategies (Lotecka & MacWhinney, 1983). Little is known regarding smokeless tobacco maintenance and cessation (see Chapter 10). Blood nicotine levels are equivalent or greater for smokeless tobacco users than for cigarette smokers (Gritz, Baer-Weiss, Benowitz, Van Vunakis, & Jarvik, 1981), and the same patterns of nicotine dependence appear to occur for both substances, including increases in use, stabilization of use, and withdrawal symptoms (Henningfield, 1986). Indeed, the need for an increased understanding of how to reduce the use of both substances in youth is imperative.

ALTERNATIVE PREVENTION AND CESSATION PROGRAM OPTIONS IN SCHOOLS

There are a variety of potential options to providing tobacco use prevention and/or cessation programming for adolescents. These include one-on-one counseling in private clinics; self-help programming involving only the child or the family; phone-based interventions; community/group programming, such as in Little Leagues, 4-H groups, and Boys and Girls Clubs; and school-based programming. School-based programming tends to be more effective than other options for at least four reasons:

1. Most youth are likely to be exposed to such programming if instituted during school hours, whereas in other contexts only a relatively small percentage of youth may be reached.
2. Schools generally are mandated by law to provide health education. Thus there is some incentive for programming.
3. Effective programming can be optimally evaluated because youth are likely to be exposed to the complete program and can generally be followed up several years postprogram.
4. Face-to-face learning is possible. The learning of both verbal and nonverbal social skills and the advantages of more personalized feedback are available within the school context.

Within the context of school programming, several options exist. These include the use of minimal or passive programming, such as posters, PA announcements, and assemblies, and the use of clinics or support groups and/or classroom-based programming. *Posters* in classrooms have the advantage of both cost- and time-effectiveness, and the likelihood of being placed in all targeted classrooms. The disadvantages with this modality are that only minimal information can be provided in a poster, and that only 25% to 50% of the students will read such a poster (Sussman, Dent, Stacy, Burton, & Flay, 1992).

School-based clinics are composed of small groups of students in which prevention or cessation information can be provided. The provision of class release time may act as an incentive to boost student recruitment (Burton, Sussman, Dent, Graham, & Hahn, 1989). High facilitator-student ratios can be reached permitting a relatively intensive intervention. The problem is that the clinic approach tends to reach relatively few students, and the attrition rate after a first session is generally approximately 50%. In spite of these disadvantages, this method may be the only face-to-face means of targeting those at the highest levels of tobacco use.

Classroom interventions provide another programming option and may be *cessation* based. The advantage of this type of intervention is that students who regularly use tobacco products—those who are not likely to be motivated to attend school-based clinics or read self-help material—are more likely to be exposed to cessation information when it is presented in a classroom setting. There are, however, several disadvantages to this approach. First, cessation material is only relevant to a relatively small subset of classroom students. Second, multisession programming is not likely to result in high cessation rates among those students for whom this programming is relevant (Burton, Sussman, Dent, et al., 1989; Pallonen, 1987). Third, provision of cessation information to adolescents can result in an expectation that continued smoking is acceptable until the necessity for cessation (i.e, development of addiction, tobacco-related health impairment, etc.) arises (Pentz, Brannon, et al., 1989).

An emphasis on classroom-based *prevention* programming, which utilizes information on the social and physical consequences of continued tobacco use, is a relatively promising option. Programming can be taught to most students of the same grade in the same year (as part of the General State Requirement [GSR] classes in the junior high school grades in the Los Angeles area), students remain a "captive" audience to tobacco education, the material is relevant to all youth because no assumption of previous tobacco use needs to be made, and the learning of new information is facilitated by face-to-face encounters.

THE PUBLIC HEALTH RESEARCHER'S PERSPECTIVE TOWARD SCHOOL-BASED PREVENTION OR CESSATION CURRICULA

The discussion that follows is based upon the experiences of the author, other health education researchers, and health educators involved in the development of school-based primary prevention or cessation curricula in research groups throughout the United States (Boyd & Glover, 1989, and Glynn, 1989, mention many of these groups). These research groups share a common perspective regarding the target population and the scope and contents of a successful curriculum. Although several definitions of the word *curriculum* have been used in the health education field and elsewhere (e.g., Anderson & Creswell, 1976; Flay et al., 1988; Kliebard, 1989; Silvestri & Flay, 1989), these primary prevention researchers generally agree that it refers to the instructional content and process of one thematic topic (e.g., smoking prevention, prevention of a sedentary lifestyle) that consists of between 5 and 20 single-hour lessons (e.g., Flay et al., 1988; Glynn, 1989; Silvestri & Flay, 1989) and can be incorporated within a semester-long health education class or clinic.

AGE OF TARGET POPULATIONS FOR TOBACCO USE PREVENTION AND CESSATION PROGRAMS

The target population for most of these health promotion/disease prevention programs is an adolescent age group (6th to 10th grade; e.g., Flay, 1985; Glynn, 1989) because risk behaviors increase dramatically during this age bracket (e.g., Lewis & Lewis, 1984; Palmer, 1970). Although a health education curriculum can be tailored to the development and skills of youth of various ages (e.g., preschool youth; Hendricks, Echols, & Nelson, 1989), and although comprehensive health education instruction begun as early as 4th grade can affect tobacco use behavior (Christenson, Gold, Katz, & Kreuter, 1985), adolescence represents a "critical period" during which the provision of an awareness of social influences and social skills training is most relevant and therefore most likely to achieve successful preventive effects (Flay, d'Avernas, Best, Kersall, & Ryan, 1983). In particular, 6th to 7th grade is the school transition period during which prevention programs appear to be most well received, whereas cessation generally is attempted among those from 9th through 12th grades.

ADVENT OF SOCIAL INFLUENCE PROGRAMS

Most of the antismoking education programs that have been developed and implemented over the years by educators and researchers at schools, voluntary health agencies, and other settings have not received the rigorous scientific evaluation necessary to judge their efficacy. Most past programs have been based on the assumption that if children know why cigarette smoking is bad for them, they will choose to not start smoking. Of those conventional smoking education programs evaluated, many have succeeded in changing students' knowledge and attitudes, but very few have consistently reduced the onset or increases of smoking behavior (Green, 1979; Thompson, 1978). As will be discussed later, such physical consequences programming is not necessarily ineffective if developed and implemented appropriately, but in a historical context most researchers perceived that such programming was ineffective. Some acknowledge that information about physical consequences programming may be effective if directed toward personally relevant consequences (Glynn, Levanthal, & Hirschman, 1985; Johnson, 1981). Most researchers have searched for alternatives to physical consequences programming.

Social influence programs that were developed beginning in 1976 were based on McGuire's work; the basic assumption was that "inoculation" to resist social pressures that serve as precipitants of use would help prevent use. This orientation showed promise, and resulting programming showed success lasting up to 3 years postprogram (Flay, 1985; Tobler, 1986).

Flay (1985) reviewed 27 school-based studies of psychosocial approaches to smoking prevention. The research studies were considered in four "generations" (presented in more detail in Chapter 3): (a) the work by Richard Evans and colleagues at the University of Houston; (b) 7 "pilot" studies of improved programs at the Universities of Stanford, Minnesota, New York, and Washington, with one school or classroom per experimental condition; (c) a third generation involving 12 improved "prototype" studies by these four groups and others, with two or three units randomly assigned to conditions; and (d) a fourth generation involving 6 studies in which maximizing internal validity was of prime concern. Reported results were fairly consistent, with each tested program seeming to reduce smoking onset by about 50%. However, none of the pilot or prototype studies considered alone provided easily interpretable results. The major contributions were improved programs and methods. The findings from the 4th generation of studies were more easily interpreted, though only 2 of them were interpreted with high confidence. Overall it seems that psychosocial approaches to smoking prevention are effective.

In summary, although traditional information-oriented programs have not been successful, comprehensive social influences programs have reduced smoking onset by as much as 50% up to 3 years postprogram. An announcement, published by the National Cancer Institute, entitled *Prevention and Cessation of Use of Smokeless Tobacco* led to the funding of several smokeless tobacco prevention studies (Boyd & Glover, 1989). The outcomes of three of these studies, which addressed both cigarette and smokeless tobacco use, appear to replicate previous findings where only use of cigarettes was considered (Elder et al., 1993; Severson et al., 1991; Sussman, Dent, Stacy, Sun, et al., 1993). Results of other smokeless tobacco prevention trials are forthcoming.

THREE

Phases in the History of School-Based Prevention Programs

Researchers have suggested that school-based prevention research should go through several progressive phases, including basic research, refinement of methodology, experimental trials, demonstration projects in large populations, and transfer of technology to diverse settings (Flay, 1986). These phases of prevention research that have formed the basis for many of the methodological and substantive components of Project TNT are discussed below.

BASIC RESEARCH

Basic research in prevention generally consists of assessment studies designed to identify the predictors of tobacco use and lead to the development of acquisition-oriented prevention programming (Chassin, Presson, & Sherman, 1985; Flay, 1986; Sussman, 1991). Basic research studies expand our understanding of one or more of the three main components of tobacco use behavior, or—to borrow a term from clinical psychology (Goldfried & Davison, 1976)—the ABCs (see Figure 3.1), where A refers to antecedents, or the variables that lead to healthy or unhealthy behavior, B refers to the behaviors, including the risk factors (seven behaviors), upon which people in

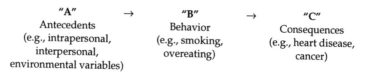

Figure 3.1. The ABCs of Health Behavior Research

the public health field tend to place a high priority (Belloc & Breslow, 1972), and C refers to consequences, defined here as "the result of something you do" (or "something that happens to you").

Using this paradigm, smoking, drinking, eating too much, driving dangerously, not exercising, sleeping irregularly or for insufficient amounts of time, stress, and poor hygiene are all classified as behaviors and may lead to such negative consequences as heart disease, cancer, or accidents. The spectrum of behaviors to be considered in health behavior research is wide and varied, and the behaviors within that spectrum tend to be interrelated (Donovan & Jessor, 1985; Sussman, Dent, Stacy, Burton, & Flay, in press).

Cancer, heart disease, and death are all consequences of tobacco use. *Morbidity* refers to quality of life, whereas *mortality* refers to longevity. Kaplan (1984) argues that both morbidity and mortality need to be taken into account to fully describe health consequences.

The first phase in developing tobacco use prevention or cessation programming (see Chapter 7 for more details) consists of assessment studies that are guided by the results of available theory. Assessment studies of tobacco use antecedents, behaviors, or perceived consequences have included several methodologies, such as the use of focus groups, interviews, questionnaires, behavioral observation, true experimental variations, and even environmental observation (e.g., refuse analysis).

As mentioned in the last chapter, recent multiple-component prevention programs based on psychosocial processes have been considered by many researchers to be the most successful at reducing the onset of risk behaviors, such as adolescent drug use, especially cigarette use (Flay, 1985; Flay et al., 1985; Glynn, 1989; Hansen, Johnson, Flay, Graham, & Sobel, 1988; Pentz, Dwyer, et al., 1989; Perry & Jessor, 1983; Silvestri & Flay, 1989). Such pro-

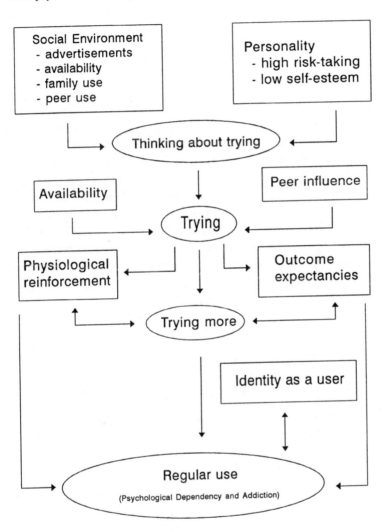

Figure 3.2. General Model of Tobacco Use Development

grams were built, in part, upon a foundation of assessment studies (e.g., as summarized by Flay et al., 1983), that helped to construct a general theoretical model of tobacco use development. A simplified model is presented as Figure 3.2.

A Model of Cigarette Smoking Development

Research has shown that those youth who smoke cigarettes (a) tend to begin smoking between the ages of 11 to 13, from both genders and from any ethnic group (African Americans may begin smoking at a slightly older age); (b) are of lower socioeconomic status than their nonsmoking peers; (c) have friends and family who are smokers; (d) are not monitored closely by family; (e) tend to be risk takers and to be relatively uninvolved with school activities; (f) tend to lack self-efficacy to resist pressures to smoke; (g) are high in perceived stress and of low self-esteem; and (h) are likely to experiment with other substances (e.g., Conrad, Flay, & Hill, 1992; Flay et al., 1983; Sussman et al., 1990; Wills, 1986). Integrating the cigarette smoking assessment study literature, Flay et al. (1983) developed a model of cigarette smoking development stages that also has been applied to the use of other substances:

1. In the first stage, the nonuser undergoes a preparation phase, in which personality, family, and peer factors operate. Risk takers, and those whose family and peers smoke, are most likely to intend to begin smoking themselves.

2. Peer social influence factors primarily operate in the second stage, during which the individual may try the substance. Frequency of direct peer pressure influences the likelihood of coping successfully through use of refusal assertion or other skills. The more frequent the influence attempt, the less likely such coping will be used successfully. Also, social images portrayed by cigarette advertisements may lead some youth to feel curious about the effects of cigarette smoking. Thus youth may gather together and smoke as a shared experience, especially if they are not closely monitored by their parents.

3. During the third stage, the individual enters into an experimental phase, in which outcome expectancies, use habits, and physiological reinforcement are shaped.

4. In the fourth and fifth stages, the adolescent becomes a regular user (i.e., using regularly every day), and physiological reinforcement, identity as a user, and addiction factors dominate as reasons for using.

These stages of development are useful because they suggest that different types of programs may be successful at preventing youth from advancing in use at different stages of use development. Most tobacco use prevention programs emphasize primary prevention and focus on counteracting social influences—addressing only the first and second stages of this model.

John Elder and colleagues recently developed an alternative model of smoking development that is based on a stages-of-change conceptualization (Stern, Prochaska, Velicer, & Elder, 1987). The three distinct components of this model are

1. Precontemplation—no desire to start smoking
2. Decision making—thinking about trying and balancing the pros and cons of smoking
3. Maintenance—smoking and increases in smoking

Although this model does not contain the theoretical richness of a model like Flay's, it is empirically rigorous. Prevention strategies could be developed, based upon the results of a questionnaire developed by this research team, to chart the tobacco use developmental stage of participating youth. Possibly this stage of acquisition model complements the comprehensive psychosocial model developed by Flay. Psychological variables tapped by Flay might best be examined as predictors of stage of acquisition (the latter might be best viewed as a dependent variable).

Who Uses Smokeless Tobacco?

Flay's model might also help to explain the development of smokeless tobacco use. Of course, more specific demographic groups (i.e., white males) are primarily associated with smokeless tobacco use, and therefore some differences in reasons for use seem likely. It is probably more accurate, therefore, to conduct separate assessment studies of smokeless tobacco product use, and to refine Flay's model and develop a more empirically supported etiological model for use with smokeless tobacco users.

Historically (since 1910), smokeless tobacco has been used by people in rural areas, such as farmers, miners, foresters, and others who work with flammable materials. Recently, however, the demographics have changed to include use by adolescent males who reside in urban as well as rural areas, widespread use among Native American males and females, and increasing use among Latino males.

Characteristically at present, smokeless tobacco users (a) are young; (b) are typically white males; (c) are involved in rigorous outdoor activities; (d) smoke cigarettes and drink alcohol (and sometimes use other drugs, but less so than smokers); (e) have friends who use, and report inflated prevalence estimates of use; (f) have fathers who use or approve of use; (g) have mothers who approve of use; (h) are from one-parent homes; (i) are favorable to a social image of being brave, athletic, hard-working, and popular; (j) believe use is fun, makes them look older and more popular, and improves sports performance; (k) believe use to be safer than smoking; (l) may be more conservative than cigarette smokers; (m) tend to prefer taking risks; (n) receive relatively poor grades; (o) endure a different pattern of effects from those who prefer ciga-rettes (i.e., a slow prolonged effect); and (p) are of a lower but more heterogenous socioeconomic (SES) background than smokers (e.g. see U.S. DHHS, 1994, chap. 4; Sussman, 1989).

It should also be remembered that there are distinctions be-tween those who use chewing tobacco and those who "dip" snuff. "Chewers" tend to be older and more distant and practical than "dippers"—who are generally younger and more outgoing and imaginative (Edmundson, Glover, Holbert, Alston, & Schroeder, 1988). Still, many similarities exist in the etiology of cigarette and smokeless tobacco use, including use among same-sexed peers involving offers or sharing of the tobacco, as well as risk-taking preferences. The etiology of the two forms of tobacco use will be described from the perspective of normative and informational social influence in the next chapter.

Caveats When Discussing Models of Tobacco Use Development

There is a tendency to study basic research as a finite process— to think linearly—and therefore to assume that once a body of knowledge of predictors of a behavior has been developed, we can move on to subsequent research steps and not have to return to earlier steps. It is not surprising, therefore, that some researchers have suggested that theoretical components testing is no longer needed in the tobacco use prevention/cessation field, or seem to suggest that basic research will not be needed at some point in the future (Glynn, 1989; Glynn & Cullen, 1989). In the history of science, however, progress is seldom linear (Boring, 1957). It is nearly always necessary to return to basic research to deal with new contexts and new innovations in theory and method. Hence research is a cyclic process—not a linear one.

It must also be remembered that only sketchy support has been documented for the types of social influence processes outlined by Flay and others. For example, recent prevention programs typically have altered many things about curricula in addition to the focus on counteracting social influence, making it difficult to ascertain if social influence is the key factor. More elaborate empirical tests of such models are still needed (Conrad et al., 1992).

THEORY-BASED EXPERIMENTAL TRIALS

Earlier on, small school-based trials were completed involving self-selection to conditions, which later became larger trials involving true field experimental designs. The evolution of this research is described by Flay (1985). Richard Evans and his colleagues at the University of Houston (Evans, 1976; Evans et al., 1978; Evans, Henderson, Hill, & Raines, 1979) derived the basis for the social influences approach, and the first tests of it are regarded as the 1st generation in Flay's review. All subsequent generations of research were influenced to varying degrees by the Houston studies.

The work on the social influences approach to smoking prevention developed by the University of Houston group relied heavily on McGuire's (1964) social inoculation theory. Social inoculation is analogous to biological inoculation, whereby a person is exposed to a small dose of an infectious agent in order to develop antibodies, thus reducing susceptibility to subsequent exposure. Applied to smoking, this model posits that resistance to persuasion will be greater if one has developed arguments with which to counteract social pressure to smoke (Evans, 1976). Two prevention studies by the Houston group (Evans et al., 1978, 1979) were based on this theory, with added theoretical bolstering from attitude change (persuasive communications) theory (McGuire, 1969) and social learning theory (Bandura, 1977).

Despite inconclusive results from the first Houston study, the theoretical derivations were firm enough to encourage other researchers to test psychosocial approaches to smoking prevention further. Seven 2nd-generation studies placed greater emphasis on elements derived from theories of social learning (Bandura, 1977), attribution (Jones et al., 1972), commitment (Kiesler, 1971), problem behavior (Jessor & Jessor, 1977), and cognitive-behavioral factors (Meichenbaum, 1977). The efficacy of peer teaching was also investigated, with theoretical reliance upon social learning theory (Hartup & Louge, 1979; Vriend, 1969).

Second-generation studies at the Universities of Stanford, Minnesota, New York, and Washington tested improved programs, with the improvements clearly derived from extant theory. The 2nd generation of research was still rather limited methodologically with only one school or classroom assigned to each experimental condition. The four groups of 2nd-generation researchers quickly moved into improved 3rd-generation studies of their approaches assigning two or three schools or classrooms per condition, usually randomly. Researchers from the Stanford and Minnesota groups were joined in 3rd-generation research by three other groups that tried the social influences approach in larger community studies (North Karelia, Oslo, and Minnesota). In addition, Shaffer and colleagues at Cambridge (Harvard Medical School) provided a 3rd-generation test of a cognitively oriented social influences curriculum, and Pentz, then at the University of Tennessee and now at the University of Southern California (USC), provided a 3rd-generation test of a general social competence skills approach to prevention.

Third-generation studies improved much on 1st- and 2nd-generation studies, including random assignment of multiple schools to conditions. However, they still exhibited many methodological problems and therefore lent themselves to several plausible alternative explanations for their findings. Most of the 3rd-generation studies are susceptible to two alternative interpretations of any observed effects. Testing-by-treatment interactions are possible because in most instances the program and data collection activities would have been perceived by students as related. Hawthorne effects are also possible in that in almost all studies program students received more special attention than controls.

The Minnesota, New York, Stanford, and USC studies attempted to test the value of various components of their programs, particularly the use of peer leaders, social versus health programs, the use of media, and the use of public commitment procedures. However, given the generally low internal validity of these studies, none of the findings from these comparisons can be accepted without further replication (Johnson, 1981; McCaul & Glasgow, 1985).

In the 4th generation of research, investigators placed increasing emphasis on maximizing internal validity. Researchers from the original Stanford (with McAlister then at Harvard) and Minnesota (with Johnson then with Hansen and Flay in Southern California) groups were responsible for improved (4th-generation) studies of the social influences approach; they were joined by four new research groups (Best, Flay, and colleagues, Canada; Fisher and colleagues in Australia; Dielman and colleagues in Michigan; and Biglan, Severson, and colleagues in Oregon). The consistency of reported results from 2nd- and 3rd-generation studies provided the impetus for improved studies. The 4th-generation studies may be characterized as large-scale field trials, with 5 or more (half with 11 or more) units (schools or classrooms) randomly assigned to each condition. Most may also be characterized as demonstration projects, summative evaluations, or efficacy trials, in that they compared only program and control conditions, without attempting to test components or providers.

All of the 4th-generation studies tested a comprehensive social influences approach. Some of the six 4th-generation studies were superior methodologically to many of the 2nd- and 3rd-generation studies. The use of simpler and more rigorous designs generally provided for greater internal validity and more interpretable findings. Nevertheless, certain methodological problems remained, and every one of the 4th-generation studies is still susceptible to one or more plausible alternative interpretations. Some of the methodological problems, such as difficulties in achieving complete random assignment, problems with program implementation, and serious attrition rates, serve to remind us of the difficulties of large-scale school-based research.

Overall, the findings from the most rigorous studies to date suggest that the social influences approach to smoking prevention can be effective. However, this conclusion seems to be tentative, given the considerable differences between studies in the patterns of reported results. Also, plausible alternative interpretations of the reported effects remain. For example, the Hawthorne effect could have occurred; students who received special attention in the classroom may have been influenced to alter their behavior or their reports of it. The likelihood of such processes causing the observed effects is small, however, especially when one considers that many tests of other approaches to smoking prevention have not reported significant effects. A more plausible alternative is that social influence curricula do not operate through traditional social influence processes but instead operate through connecting social cues to whatever information is provided. Such a cue effect is consistent with the view that prevention information must be tied to "high-risk" situations for it to become accessible from memory. Accessibility, in turn, is necessary for any behavioral effects (Stacy, Dent, et al., 1990; Stacy, MacKinnon, & Pentz, 1993; Stacy, Widaman, & Marlatt, 1990), consistent with most theories of memory. Accessibility is an example of the factors that may correlate with the provision of "social influence" curricula in an uncontrolled manner. Additional theory-based research is needed to more fully explore such factors.

USE OF PROGRAMS OF PROVEN EFFECTIVENESS WITH LARGE DEFINED POPULATIONS

A next step among national researchers has been to demonstrate that successful programs from smaller environments are adaptable to larger populations (e.g., urban youth in major cities) and that these programs can be replicated nationally. National Cancer Institute (NCI)-funded tobacco control Projects COMMIT and ASSIST, as well as multiple projects funded in California through Proposition 99 monies, are examples of this ongoing research.

Novotny, Romano, Davis, and Mills (1992) outlined sev‹
elements of current tobacco use prevention and contro
aimed at large populations by NCI and others. These ele‹

1. *Surveillance* of tobacco-related knowledge, beliefs, and behavior among adults and adolescents of various subgroups
2. *Problem assessments,* including pattern of tobacco use, intervention access, and disease impact
3. *Legislation and policies* to refocus tobacco use as a public health concern, which includes implementation of clean-indoor-air policies, restrictions on access to tobacco by minors, restrictions on advertising, and tax increases
4. *Health department and community-based programs,* including Projects COMMIT and ASSIST, and several NCI intervention trials
5. *Public information campaigns,* including the use of social marketing techniques, provision of behavior change information, and utilization of statewide media campaigns, such as are used in California
6. *Technical information collection and dissemination,* including the use of abstracting services and dissemination of prevention and cessation manuals and materials to state and local health departments
7. *Coalition building,* such as the creation of advisory boards of community action groups to lobby for antitobacco legislation or to facilitate the dissemination of prevention and cessation materials

Novotny et al. (1992) conclude by asserting that multifaceted public health activities for controlling tobacco use need continuous assessment and evaluation in order to adapt them to different contexts—a conclusion consistent with Sussman (1991).

Research with large defined populations presents a number of challenges, generally including (a) the need to involve community leaders and to establish community ownership in order to maximize implementation within a site; (b) the need to approximate equivalent implementation across large sites or regions of the country; and (c) the ability to disseminate successful research.

The first challenge is particularly critical because research demonstrates that communities are far more likely to carry out new programs when there is a feeling of belonging or ownership (Pentz, 1986). On the other hand, when relevant "gatekeepers" resist the research and either change or reduce the programs, program success and/or effectiveness can be diminished considerably. The second challenge, approximating equivalent implementation across large areas, may be quite difficult because geography and demographics vary considerably across the country. A program that is highly generalizable, however, should replicate across similar contexts (e.g., schools). The third challenge can be overcome if a community will adopt a program, send its messages throughout the system, and reinvent or alter the program while maintaining its key elements for different contexts. Ongoing research is attempting to find new ways to overcome these challenges. The issue of technology transfer also is addressed in Chapter 13 of this book.

GENERALIZATION OF PROGRAMMING TO SPECIAL POPULATIONS OR NEW PROBLEM AREAS: PROJECT TNT

Still more theoretical testing has been supported by NCI, particularly with special populations (e.g., minorities) or regarding new problem areas (e.g., smoke-free tobacco products). Project Towards No Tobacco Use (Project TNT) was designed, in part, to learn more about the social influence processes that previous research has shown may govern cigarette smoking onset, prevention, and cessation—and how these processes may apply to smokeless tobacco use. Project TNT, therefore, can be considered a direct outgrowth of the work instigated by Evans and colleagues. The prevention component of this project sampled over 7,000 students from 29 different school districts in southern California. The cessation component sampled (including surveys) over 3,000 students from 22 different school districts in California and Illinois.

In the prevention component, Project TNT evaluated the relative effectiveness of normative versus informational social-influence-derived tobacco use prevention programming. As outlined in Chapter 4, these aspects of social influence are seen as two of the major mediators of social-influence-oriented tobacco use prevention programs.

In the cessation component, Project TNT assessed the relative effectiveness of addiction- versus psychosocial-oriented cessation programming. As outlined in Chapter 13, these are two of the primary types of alternative programming that can be used to intervene on the regular use of tobacco by adolescents.

For both components, the program of research consisted of four phases. These phases were designed to enhance understanding of tobacco use etiology and measurement, develop theoretically based curricula, and effectively implement and evaluate the programs. These four phases were

1. Seven assessment studies that extended the adolescent tobacco use knowledge base (in etiology and measurement) from cigarettes to smokeless tobacco
2. A large-scale longitudinal self-report study among half of the junior high school students, as well as use of grade cohort-level repeated measurements among some junior high schools and high schools
3. A 1-year, empirically linked, prevention curricula development process and a 2-year cessation recruitment and curricula development process
4. Implementation of the prevention and cessation curricula, with a 2-year follow-up of the prevention curricula and a 3-month follow-up of the cessation curricula

The etiology and measurement studies will be summarized in Part Two of this book, with a special focus on their relevance for various issues in adolescent tobacco use prevention. Part Three will describe curricula development, implementation, and evaluation of the prevention trial. Part Four will describe the recruitment protocol and curricula development, implementation, and evaluation of the cessation trial.

Project TNT has built upon past research in school-based tobacco use prevention by testing components of previously successful comprehensive social influences prevention programs. Project TNT has also expanded on previous adolescent prevention programming by developing a more state-of-the-art physical consequences curriculum as a single-component comparison curriculum. Finally, Project TNT has expanded on previous adolescent cessation programming by providing a large-scale experimental test of alternative high school clinic cessation programs.

PART TWO

Theoretical Basis and Methodological Considerations of the Prevention Component of Project Towards No Tobacco Use (Project TNT)

Part Two provides the theoretical basis of Project TNT. In Chapter 4, the theoretical underpinnings for an experimental test of the two major types of social influence are presented: that is, normative social influence and informational social influence. Theory in Chapter 4 integrates variables first described in Part One (e.g., Flay's model) within one or the other of these two types of social influence. In addition, material on physical consequences often is contained in social influences curricula, and the theoretical issues involved in the use of this material is discussed. Thus Chapter 4 makes the reader familiar with the ways that concepts were manipulated as different classroom curricula in Project TNT. Part Two also provides the methodological backbone of Project TNT. Chapter 5 presents the recruitment procedure, issues of human subjects' consent, and how different confounds and attrition were controlled for. In Chapter 6, methods of assessing student tobacco use are discussed, including biochemical validation, school and store personnel interviews, refuse analysis, and naturalistic observation.

Social Influence in Etiology and Prevention of Tobacco Use

Suggestive evidence for social psychological causes of trial and regular use of cigarettes is prolific (e.g., Chassin, Presson, & Sherman, 1990; Conrad et al., 1992; Flay et al., 1983). Most adolescents experiment with tobacco in a social context with friends of the same sex (Bewley, Bland, & Harris, 1974; Friedman, Lichtenstein, & Biglan, 1985; Palmer, 1970). Although much of the evidence cannot yet disentangle whether people pick similar (tobacco-using) friends or whether they are influenced by these friends, adolescent social group influences may be the most important precipitants of tobacco use. Adolescent social group influence varies by type of pressure exerted (Eiser, 1985).

A group often wants its members to act and believe as members of the rest of the group do. *Social influence* is a general term for the many psychological effects that others have on an individual. Social psychology researchers have noted that there are two main types of pressure that a group exerts on its members (Deutsch & Gerard, 1955; Kelley, 1952; Kiesler & Kiesler, 1970). First, the group may want its members to act in ways consistent with the group in order to gain or maintain acceptance of other group members; the group applies a *normative* social influence on the person. Second, the group may want its members to share similar attitudes regarding the social meanings and frequencies of different behaviors; the group applies an *informational* social influence on the person. Although several theories have been used to study the etiology and prevention of tobacco use, including various informational, affective, cognitive-behavioral, and life skills models (U.S. DHHS, 1991b, chap. 4), Project TNT employed concepts from classical social psychology literature to delineate two main etiological variables (some of the material here is adapted from Sussman, 1989). Many of the other theories of tobacco use etiology are compatible with aspects of one or both of these two social psychological domains. We believe that this two-component model provides a heuristic function by summarizing or simplifying many labels of social influence within a two-category scheme.

NORMATIVE SOCIAL INFLUENCE

Definition

Adolescent groups want their members to comply with certain standards of behavior, which may include participating regularly in group activities, giving in to "dares," and providing social support to other group members (e.g., Johnson, 1980; Larkin, 1979; Lewis & Lewis, 1984; Sussman, Dent, Raynor, et al., 1988). In turn, groups provide social reinforcers to indicate acceptance of compliant group members (e.g., Wills, 1985) that include companionship and instrumental support (group members will spend time with the individual and help the individual with practical needs), affection (group members will express liking of the individual), and status (others will place the individual in a valued position within the group).

Normative social influence is likely to have a greater impact when the following conditions exist: (a) explicit behaviors are desired by the group; (b) explicit reinforcers are given in return for performing those behaviors; (c) behavior-relevant information is widely disseminated, allowing the group to serve less as an information source; (d) the group has little information regarding the individual's true opinions; (e) the self-presentation skills of the individual are high; and (f) negative consequences for not conforming are reliable.

Cigarette Smoking

In the context of tobacco use, normative social influence is likely to have a greater impact among those young persons who have enough information to feel apprehensive about the negative physical and social consequences of using tobacco but who yield to offers of tobacco to gain acceptance by the group. Several research results support this influence of normative social influence on cigarette smoking. Most youth refer to initial cigarette smoking as an unexpected event beginning with an offer from someone else that in many cases resulted in verbally aversive behavior if the youth did not try the cigarette (Friedman et al., 1985). Self-reported difficulty in refusing cigarette offers from one's peer group has been found to be a stronger predictor of future cigarette smoking behavior than peer smoking in Israeli youth (Salomon, Stein, Eisenberg, & Klein, 1984). This difficulty has also been found to be a better predictor than intentions to smoke in the future of subsequent trial of cigarettes one year later across ethnic groups in a large Los Angeles-area sample (Sussman, Dent, Flay, Hansen, & Johnson, 1987). Youth who are likely to use cigarettes are those who also show inadequate refusal assertion skills—who tend to respond passively (e.g., "hedge"), rather than assertively, to cigarette offers (Hops et al., 1986; Reardon, Sussman, & Flay, 1989). Cigarette smoking prevention programs that focus in part on teaching assertive refusal skills and motivating young people to resist normative social influences have been successful in preventing cigarette smoking (Flay, 1985).

Smokeless Tobacco Use

In the recent past, it is likely that informational social influence prevailed as a determinant of smokeless tobacco use. However, smokeless tobacco use continues to spread from rural areas (traditionally associated with smokeless tobacco use) to urban areas (Boyd & Associates, 1987). Urban areas contain fewer adult role models who use smokeless tobacco and fewer values historically associated with smokeless tobacco. Thus normative social influence may become relatively more dominant as the precipitant of smokeless tobacco use (e.g., Brubaker & Loftin, 1987). In addition, smokeless tobacco may now be viewed as one of several substances used by youth as "dares," in which normative social influence predominates (Hu, in preparation; Simon et al., 1993).

INFORMATIONAL SOCIAL INFLUENCE

Definition

Adolescence is the major life period during which the individual's self-identity develops (Erickson, 1968; Jessor, 1984). The adolescent is faced with rapid life changes (e.g., entry into junior high and high school), encounters new opportunities (e.g., team sports, jobs), and learns much information about his or her social world. Adolescent groups play a major role in this process (Brown & Lohr, 1987; Erickson, 1968; Jessor, 1984; Jessor & Jessor, 1977; Lewis & Lewis, 1984). Groups provide (a) definitions of and information about social reality, and (b) evaluation or validation of the individual's own opinions, which motivates private acceptance of group standards of behavior (Ajzen & Fishbein, 1970; Bandura, 1977; Festinger, 1954; Kiesler & Kiesler, 1970).

Three examples of the effects of informational social influence include one's identification with social images, estimates of prevalence of a behavior, and perspective regarding an evaluative quality of a behavior. First, the group defines those social images to which its members aspire. Identification with group social images, which include appearing independent, mature or grown-up, tough, exciting, or gregarious, is associated with cigarette smoking and smokeless tobacco use (Baumrind, 1985; Botvin & Eng, 1979; Botvin & Wills, 1985; Burton, Sussman, Hansen, Johnson, & Flay, 1989; Chassin, Presson, Sherman, & Margolis, 1988; Dent, Sussman,

Johnson, Hansen, & Flay, 1987; Elder & Stern, 1986; Flay et al., 1983; McAlister, 1983; McCarthy, 1985; Newman, 1984; Salomon et al., 1984). Second, the group may suggest that "everyone uses tobacco." Those who hold inflated prevalence estimates of use may then perceive that tobacco use is a routine behavior among their peers or adults. This social information may influence one's own future behavior. Relatively inflated prevalence estimates of smoking are among the best prospective psychosocial predictors of trial and increases in smoking (Chassin et al., 1984; Collins et al., 1987; Sussman, Dent, Mestel-Rauch, et al., 1988). Likewise, smokeless tobacco users give higher prevalence estimates of its use than do nonusers (Chassin, Presson, Shermon, McLaughlin, & Goila, 1985).

Third, the group defines the range of opinion within which an individual conforms. Perspective Theory research indicates a separation between the individual's self-ratings on an attitude scale and his or her content position ratings regarding a specific behavior (Ostrom & Upshaw, 1968; Upshaw & Ostrom, 1984). Many young persons' self-ratings (e.g., that they are "good people" or hold "moderate opinions") are less strongly anchored to specific attitude content (e.g., that they believe in one's right to use tobacco in public) than are adults' ratings because they are at that stage of life when their self-identities are forming. Content positions they identify with and adhere to are strongly influenced by peer group values and beliefs. When they associate with a new peer group, their range of available content alternatives is likely to expand or contract, which could lead to a change in their content positions but not their global self-ratings. For example, new members of a group may feel that their opinions and behaviors are appropriate because they maintain a moderate stance within the group. Yet the more extreme the reference group's opinions are, the more extreme the opinions of a moderate new group member may become. By associating within relatively deviant groups, a young person who identifies him or herself as being a moderate person is likely also to hold opinions favorable toward tobacco use.

Several studies have been completed in various experimental and nonexperimental contexts to discern the conditions under which group information is likely to *influence its members' opinions* (e.g., Deutsch & Gerard, 1955; Eiser, 1980; Gottlieb, 1985; Hall &

Wellman, 1985; Kiesler & Kiesler, 1970). Generally, these studies found that a person is more likely to come to believe the information presented by the group when he or she (a) is less certain about his or her own opinions, (b) has less access to alternative information, and (c) perceives that the group obtains success in various situations. Unanimous agreement within the group also will enhance its informational influence on new members (e.g., Allen & Wilder, 1980).

In addition, youth who are unable to make social ties with new peers to obtain competing social information are more likely to be subject to informational social influence (Granovetter, 1973). Two variables inhibit making such ties: (a) membership in a social network that exerts much informational social influence over the individual (e.g., on a day-to-day basis), and (b) inadequate skills necessary to make social ties with new people.

Cigarette Smoking

Informational influence on cigarette smoking development is likely to have a greater impact in social contexts where much smoking is occurring and being observed, and where information regarding alternatives to smoking is relatively less salient as is often the case in some lower socioeconomic groups (e.g., Eckert, 1983, 1989; Flay et al., 1983; Semmer, Cleary, Dwyer, Fuchs, & Lippert, 1987). For example, in Eckert's (1983) participant observation study of tobacco use in different sociocultural groups of youth at a Michigan high school, two major groups were evident: "burnouts" and "jocks/populars." Burnouts were defined as a community of youth who were directed toward working-class lives, saw a continuity in their lives from high school to adulthood, were neighborhood oriented, and learned to share cigarettes and personal belongings in a tight-knit (high-density) community of other burnouts. Jocks/populars were defined as a relatively loose-knit community of college-bound, middle-class youth who were future directed, involved in various school activities, and disinclined to smoke. Jocks/populars were also more mobile and possessed conversational skills that enabled them to interact with persons from other groups and to choose alternatives to smoking.

Smokeless Tobacco Use

Given current trends toward increased smokeless tobacco use and away from cigarette use among male youth (e.g., Hunter et al., 1986), it is imperative to understand why smokeless tobacco is being used. Most reasons that have been suggested as contributors to the rise in smokeless tobacco use are informational social influence oriented. These reasons could be learned through direct instruction or by watching others. They include (a) media campaigns that employ well-known athletes to teach people how to use smokeless tobacco and to model its use (e.g., Christen & Swanson, 1983; Ernster, 1989; Jones, 1987); (b) the belief that smokeless tobacco use is a safe alternative to cigarette smoking (e.g., Lichtenstein, Severson, Friedman, & Ary, 1984); (c) the belief that smokeless tobacco is more convenient to use than cigarettes (e.g., no matches are needed, it is easy to conceal, and it is inexpensive); and (d) a specific social image associated with use of smokeless tobacco versus cigarettes among males (e.g., Chassin, Presson, Sherman, McLaughlin, & Goila, 1985; Chassin et al., 1988). The smokeless tobacco user is seen as being relatively hardworking, courageous, and athletic (Chassin, Presson, Sherman, McLaughlin, & Goila, 1985; Chassin et al., 1988). This social image may be quite appealing to some adolescent males, but not to others.

Several studies indicate that chewing and dipping occurs almost solely among males (e.g., Boyd & Associates, 1987). Christen (1976) and Glover, Christen, and Henderson (1981) reported anecdotal data from adolescents confirming that one reason to use smokeless tobacco is to look "macho." Displaying a faded snuff can mark on the rear pocket of blue jeans, for example, signals a "macho" image to peers. This may be considered an informational social influence because youth learn an associative tie between a social image and tobacco use, and many youth do not report that social acceptability would result from that image. Rather, they are trying to match their own self-image and their ideal self-image to this tobacco-use-related social image (Burton, Sussman, Hansen, et al., 1989). Sex typing related to images portrayed in smokeless tobacco advertisements help explain sex differences in use of this product, as well as the fact that most smokeless tobacco products involve "spitting," an activity that females generally do not enjoy (Gritz, Ksir, & McCarthy, 1985).

COUNTERING NORMATIVE AND INFORMATIONAL INFLUENCES

There are three major ways that people can be taught to reduce group pressures to use tobacco. First, youth can be taught to try to maintain their status quo within the group while not conforming to group influences to use tobacco. Indeed, a large minority of youth who belong to tobacco-using groups are not users themselves (Sussman, Dent, Simon, et al., 1993). Second, they can learn to withdraw from the behavioral demands or informational control of the group. Third, they can learn to assert themselves within the group and try to persuade others not to use tobacco. The goal of a normative social influence program is to counteract group pressures on the individual to achieve group acceptance by using tobacco, whereas the goal of an informational social influence program is to counteract pressures to adopt attitudes and values favorable to tobacco use. One can combat normative or informational social influences by learning strategies that lead one to maintain one's status quo in the group, withdraw from the group, or act on the group.

Countering Normative Social Influence

Maintaining the Status Quo

One can learn to maintain acceptance from the group in various ways without agreeing to use tobacco. Ingratiation Theory suggests a means of accomplishing such a stance (Jones, 1964; Jones & Wortman, 1973). Ingratiation Theory posits that one will be even more liked by group members if one disagrees on unimportant points but agrees with the group on more important points, than if one agrees with everything (in which case one may appear to be a "yes" person). Thus if one disagrees about the acceptability of using tobacco but provides a lot of rewards to the group (e.g., expresses affection, is a good listener), one may be able to maintain the group's affection even while not using tobacco.

It is possible that the group accepts nonusers even if the principles of Ingratiation Theory are not applied. The use of cognitive restructuring techniques can help youth modify inner speech consistent with using tobacco in a situation. For example, youth can practice changing inner speech such as "I won't be accepted by the group if I don't use" to "I will still be accepted by the group whether I use tobacco or not" (Schinke & Gilchrist, 1985).

Distancing

Youth can withdraw from the behavior demands of groups in several ways. Simply avoiding or escaping from high-risk situations is a way of withdrawing from group demands. Self-instructional training and stress inoculation training procedures (Meichenbaum, 1977, 1985) are also relevant to preventing normative conformity processes, which help young people to distance themselves from the group and its acceptance demands. These strategies (a) help the individual to become more aware of impending situations and behaviors that increase the probability of yielding to tobacco offers, and (b) provide the person with self-statements that serve to cue them to avoid an immediately threatening situation, to invoke an appropriate refusal strategy when the high-risk situation is not avoidable, and to mentally rehearse coping with negative affect that could result from being exposed to such situations (Meichenbaum, 1985).

Perhaps normative social influence is best combated by teaching refusal assertion skills. Refusal assertion techniques help one to reject explicit behavioral demands of a group. Often these techniques are used as a means to teach one how to leave an aversive social situation skillfully. Still, the type of refusal assertion training program that would be most helpful to youth depends on what mediates the refusal skill deficit: that is, the most appropriate instruction is contingent on whether the deficit is learning or performance based (Bellack & Hersen, 1977; Gambrill & Richey, 1975; Kelly, 1982). A recent experimental study suggests that refusal assertion deficits are based on both learning and performance but not on motivation (Turner et al., 1993; see also Chapter 7 of this book).

Acting on the Group

Some refusal assertion techniques act to change norms regarding those behaviors that have been serving as criteria of group acceptance. The refusal assertion technique "strength in numbers" posits that refusal assertion will be more effective, and will tend to alter group norms, if the person has a friend along who will also say "no." The refusal assertion technique often called "reversing the pressure" is one where the offeree directly acts on the group to change norms. For example, the youth who is pressured to use tobacco indicates to the offerer that to maintain his or her acceptance, the tobacco offer should be withdrawn.

More importantly, the zeitgeist in tobacco use prevention research is changing. In an effort to reach the Surgeon General's goal of achieving a smoke-free young America by the year 2000 (Koop, 1986), more attempts are being made to expediently change the tobacco use "social milieu." To change the general social acceptability of tobacco use, researchers are placing an increased emphasis on the use of social activism in the community (Perry & Jessor, 1983) and on legislative constraints. Activism activities may include tobacco butt cleanup campaigns at schools, "Just Say No" clubs and banners, or attempts to instill the acceptability of broad-based healthy lifestyles ("wellness") instead of just focusing on tobacco use per se (Perry & Jessor, 1983). The use of legislative constraints provides a passive means of protecting the community's health such as limiting the availability of tobacco products. Wallack (1984) suggests that such a health protection perspective provides a more effective means of enhancing health outcomes than do strategies based on the individual. This perspective not only provides a passive means of controlling tobacco use but also expresses widespread social disapproval of tobacco use and may provide both normative and informational influences on behavior.

Countering Informational Social Influence

Maintaining the Status Quo

One can maintain status quo within the group, in terms of total amount of shared values and beliefs, while not using tobacco. This can be accomplished if one is taught how to search for new areas of mutual interest with group members, or how to explore more deeply the areas of established mutual interest that do not include tobacco use.

One can also combat informational influences by finding alternative means of conforming to social image pressures, such as pressures to act like an adult or seek excitement. Alternatives programs may include athletic risk-taking activities such as hill climbing and skiing (Swisher & Hu, 1983). Alternatively, simply asserting that one already has a certain social image (e.g., is mature) through participation in other activities (e.g., having a job), and that tobacco use would not serve to further enhance this image, could serve to help maintain that individual's social image within the group (e.g., Upshaw & Ostrom, 1984).

Distancing

One can reduce reliance on the group for information by learning problem solving and conversational skills to meet new people so that one processes competing information (e.g., Botvin & Eng, 1979; Botvin & Wills, 1985). Skills training should be combined with social image modification. Being confronted with prevalent same-aged adolescent social values, the individual should change his or her health-related social values and use newly learned social skills in a healthful direction (Kristiansen, 1986; Rokeach, 1973; Schwartz & Inbar-Saban, 1988). Direct instruction of youth regarding awareness of peer, family, advertisement, and entertainment informational influences and provision of accurate prevalence estimates of tobacco use also allow the individual to better understand determinants of his or her own behavior and allow him or her to select new, prosocial behaviors.

Acting on the Group

Youth can be taught to act on the group by providing corrective information. One method of modifying informational social influence to use drugs was tested in a program that changed information regarding alcohol use (Alcohol Abuse Prevention Trial [Project AAPT]; Hansen & Graham, 1991; Hansen, Graham, et al., 1988). In this method, youth stand under signs that indicate their opinions of the social image of a drinker, for example, and the class is confronted with the low prevalence and lack of agreement regarding types of social images associated with use. These strategies would seem to apply to tobacco use as well.

STUDIES ON SOCIAL INFLUENCE
IN THE PROJECT POPULATION

Several studies that investigated issues of relevance to theories of social influence in adolescent tobacco use were conducted by Project TNT. Two of these studies, the Group Names Study and the Social Influence in an Interactional Perspective Study, are described in this section. Social influence as a multidimensional predictor of tobacco use and our rationale for using a two-factor model of social influence (as opposed to a more complicated model) also are discussed. Additional Project TNT studies that have relevance to social influence are described in subsequent chapters. These include studies that were primarily designed as methodology studies, as outlined in Chapter 6, as well as a study on refusal assertion content in curricula, as outlined in Chapter 7.

The Group Names Study

The Group Names Study (Sussman et al., 1990) investigated the possibility that self-reported student peer group membership, and reports of student groups in general, discriminated tobacco users from nonusers. The study was conducted to obtain more information about student groups that use tobacco, in order to obtain more knowledge about the normative and informational social influences that underlie membership in particular student groups. In general, youth who engage in cigarette and other drug use report problem-prone feelings and values, including low self-esteem, noninvolvement with school and poor grades, and high risk-taking preferences (e.g., Jessor & Jessor, 1977). Mosbach and Leventhal (1988) provided the first empirically based investigation of tobacco use and problem-prone values among discrete adolescent groups. Using a self-report group identification approach adapted from Brown and Trujillo (1985), they classified four major groups among a sample of 341 seventh and eighth graders from a Wisconsin junior high school: "hot-shots," "regulars," "jocks," and "dirts." "Hot-shots," or popular kids, were described as leaders in academic activities and scored in the midrange among the groups in self-reported risk taking and self-esteem. "Regulars" were described as normal or typical of their grade; they scored the lowest in risk taking and the highest in self-esteem. "Jocks" were described as having a strong interest in team and individual sports activities, and they scored somewhat low on both risk taking and self-esteem. Finally, the "dirts" (to whom subsequently we will refer as the "high-risk" youth) were described in terms of problem behaviors including smoking, drinking, and doing poorly at school; they scored highest on risk taking and in the midrange among the other groups in self-esteem.

These researchers found that although two of the groups, the high-risk youth ("dirts") and the "hot-shots," composed 15% of the total sample, they accounted for 56% of the smokers. High-risk youth ("dirts") were the most likely to use cigarettes. They were similar to that type of youth portrayed by problem behavior theory; however, they were not the lowest in self-esteem and were moderately satisfied with their lives. "Hot-shots" were academically and socially successful youth who seemed to be dissatisfied with their achievements and who desired greater social acceptance. It may be surprising that a group not usually considered to be problem prone would show such a high rate of tobacco use.

Unfortunately, the Mosbach and Leventhal study did not assess group differences in the use of smokeless tobacco; the "jocks," another group often not considered to be problem prone and whose group definition is one of being athletic, might be most likely to use smokeless tobacco. In Sussman et al. (1990), we performed a replication study using the same group definitions as Mosbach and Leventhal to classify adolescents into groups. The sample from whom we obtained completed questionnaires consisted of 340 seventh-grade students from three public junior high schools and 615 tenth-grade students from two public high schools, representing 77% of all the 7th- and 10th-grade students enrolled at the five schools. The schools were selected to balance the sample on region, ethnicity, and gender variables.

The present study replicated several of Mosbach and Leventhal's results with a sample of southern California adolescents. For the most part, the same types of groups were identified, and our groups varied in ways consistent with the earlier findings regarding tobacco and other drug use, activities, and personal attributes. We did identify a 5th group, "skaters," who were somewhat high in risk taking and reported interest in an outdoor skateboarding activity. In our study, high-risk youth were most likely to smoke cigarettes. In addition, they were most likely to report experimentation with different drugs, were higher than all other groups in risk taking, and were the lowest in grade point average. Contrary to their results, but consistent with other research, we did find high-risk youth to be lowest in self-esteem. We also found that the "hot-shots" were least likely among the groups to be smokers. Contrary to our prediction, we found that skaters and high-risk youth were more likely to be current users of smokeless tobacco than were "jocks." Our data suggest that both forms of tobacco are used by problem-prone youth. We speculate that high-risk adolescent groups most likely to use smokeless tobacco products are involved in risky and physically vigorous outdoor activities, away from adult supervision, that (a) allow easier access to "spitting" tobacco juice, (b) preclude experimentation with hard drugs to be able to achieve satisfactory performance, and (c) may result in slightly higher self-esteem for achieving good performance.

In summary, risk for tobacco use can be revealed by self-identified group membership, which, consistent with previous research (e.g., Jessor & Jessor, 1977), generally includes problem-prone attributes of poor school performance, low self-esteem, and high risk taking.

Membership in one group versus another may reflect different behavioral methods of achieving common developmental goals of social identity and independence (Brown & Lohr, 1987). Tobacco-using youth appear to have fewer ties to, or are blocked from, conventional goals and behavior, and they may search for alternative ways to achieve these goals. These alternative behaviors often are problem prone and appear to vary in extremity of deviance depending, in part, on specific performance demands of the activity engaged in. It is likely that both normative and informational social influences operate among these youth regarding both cigarette smoking and smokeless tobacco use. Perceived social images sought after through group self-identification certainly are related to informational social influence, whereas it is likely that maintaining group acceptance in such groups involves yielding to normative pressures to participate in activities such as tobacco use.

Subsequent work has identified use of closed-ended group names categories as prospective predictors of tobacco use one year later (Sussman, Dent, McAdams, et al., 1994). "Group names" is a good psychosocial prospective predictor of tobacco use among young adolescents. It summarizes social influences not captured by other variables, such as peer tobacco use or peer approval of tobacco use.

Social Influence in an Interactional Perspective

Few studies have examined the relevance of social-influence-related moderator variables in the genesis of adolescent smoking. In Stacy, Sussman, Dent, Burton, and Flay (1992), the interactive effects of moderator variables with social influence (peer smoking and peer approval) on adolescent smoking were examined in a sample of high school students. Potential moderator variables of the effects of social influence were self-efficacy judgments, self-esteem, perceived stress, parental supervision after school, and gender. Results demonstrated that self-efficacy judgments (regarding ability to resist social pressures) significantly moderated the predictive effects of social influence on smoking tendencies.

That is, greater self-efficacy *decreased* the effect of social influence on behavior. These findings are consistent with theories suggesting that certain personality or situational variables act as buffers that either protect the adolescent against social influence or make the adolescent more susceptible to such influence. This "moderator" approach is in marked contrast to approaches in which self-efficacy is either another additive (direct-effect) predictor or a mediator of tobacco use. In these latter approaches, self-efficacy (regarding social pressure) should have an influence even among those without any social pressures to smoke. In the opinion of the present authors, this view has not been well justified theoretically.

Social Influence as a Multidimensional Predictor of Tobacco Use

Several theoretical and empirical studies have shown social influence constructs to be empirically separable and predictive of tobacco use (Sussman, 1989). Two examples of this work include that completed by Stacy, Sussman, Hansen, Johnson, and Flay (1993) and Graham, Marks, and Hansen (1991). Stacy, Sussman, et al. (1993) examined psychosocial predictors of smoking onset in a 2-year prospective study involving 1,116 adolescents. The effects of social influence variables were investigated before the subjects' own smoking behavior could affect the social influence variables themselves, for subjects were followed longitudinally before smoking onset until many subjects had become smokers 2 years later (in 9th grade). Covariance structure analysis revealed discriminant validity and differential predictive validity for six distinct social influence constructs: perceived susceptibility to direct social influence, perceived peer approval for use, number of direct offers, prevalence overestimates of smoking, friends' smoking, and tobacco use social image perceptions. Results indicated a predictive precedence of susceptibility to direct social influence, peer approval for smoking, and prevalence estimates. Specifically, perceived peer approval for smoking and susceptibility to direct offers to use tobacco, in an informational milieu that suggests widespread peer use, led adolescents to begin and continue to smoke, regardless of (a) number of direct tobacco offers made, (b) reports of friends' smoking, or (c) the tobacco use social image expectancies these adolescents held in 7th grade. These results suggested that perceived peer approval for use, along with incorrect information regarding smoking prevalence among same-aged others, will lead youths to succumb to the first tobacco offers made to them by friends or other smokers even if they hold negative tobacco use social image expectancies. This study lent etiological support to other studies that found the normative social influence variable of peer approval to be the major mediator of successful social influence program effects (e.g., MacKinnon et al., 1991), and provided partial empirical support to the picture of primary prevention suggested in "Just Say No" campaigns. This study also did lend support to one informational social influence variable, inflated prevalence estimates (e.g., Sussman, Dent, Raynor, et al., 1988). Dares to use tobacco, within a perceived context in which much tobacco use occurs, are likely to decrease one's self-efficacy to refuse offers, enhance one's sense of social influence "out there" to use tobacco, and thus maximize one's yielding to offers or temptation to use tobacco (Dr. William B. Hansen, personal communication).

Graham et al. (1991) examined psychosocial predictors of recent alcohol and cigarette use in a one-year prospective study involving 526 adolescents. The results of their study supported their hypothesized model positing three distinct social influence processes underlying adolescent alcohol and cigarette use: (a) active pressure involving explicit offers to try alcohol or tobacco; (b) passive pressure involving social modeling; and (c) overestimation of peer use. They argue that past research on the causes of drug use onset and experimentation in adolescents has treated social influence as a single, broadly defined concept. Their results showed that at least three types of social influence can be identified, each with a significant, unique effect on future substance use.

Both the Stacy, Sussman, et al. (1993) and Graham et al. (1991) studies support the perspective that the term *social influence* refers to more than one process. In Project TNT, we studied social influence as two processes, normative and informational social influence, based on earlier basic social psychology research (Deutch & Gerard, 1955). Direct tobacco use offers and peer approval for use are main normative social influence constructs. Prevalence of use overestimates, social image perceptions, and friends use are main informational social influence constructs. The Project TNT curricula, which separate informational and normative social influence, are presented in more detail in Chapter 8.

Limitations of and Rationale for the Social Influences Conception

This normative-informational dichotomy is only one of several ways to conceptualize psychosocial influences on tobacco use. There are at least *four limitations* one should consider when using these two elements of social influence as a research or intervention guide. First, discriminant validity between the two types of social influence has not always been achieved (e.g., Stacy et al., 1992). Second, more than two general factors sometimes are found (e.g., Stacy, Sussman, et al., 1993). Third, one may regard these two types of social influence as inevitably combined. For example, from a subjective expected utility perspective (Flay et al., 1988, p. 588), informational social influence might be viewed as perceptions of likelihoods, or *expectancies,* such as the prevalence of tobacco use or the likelihood that tobacco use would lead one to achieve a certain social image. Normative social influence might be viewed as a perception of the social *value* to be obtained by using tobacco, such as peer acceptance. An averaging of social influence expectancies and values may reflect a single social cognitive process that ultimately leads to tobacco use behavior. Finally, this normative-informational theoretical formulation partially overlaps with other models of tobacco use development, including that of Flay (Flay et al., 1983) and Ajzen and Fishbein (1970). (For a summary of other theoretical notions such as various social cognitive, social learning, social bonding, intrapersonal, and multivariate models, see Petraitis, Flay, and Miller, 1994, and Conrad et al., 1992.) In the theory of reasoned action (Ajzen & Fishbein, 1970, 1980), perceived social norms and attitudes toward a behavior combine to elicit behavioral intentions and subsequent behavior. The attitude component of this model may reflect informational social influence, whereas the subjective norms component may reflect normative social influence.

The rationale for using the present two-component perspective involves both theoretical and pragmatic decisions. First, the distinction between normative and informational social influence as applied to tobacco use prevention was derived from basic social psychology research (Deutsch & Gerard, 1955; Kiesler & Kiesler, 1970), has been suggested by several researchers (e.g., Eiser, 1985; Evans, 1988; Sussman, 1989), and has been empirically supported in recent research studies (e.g., Cialdini, Reno, & Kallgren, 1990; Graham et al., 1991). For example, Cialdini and colleagues have demonstrated experimentally that subjects will act on informational or normative social cues differentially based on manipulation of both the subjects' focus of attention and salience of the cue. Thus there is reasonable theoretical and empirical support for this conception.

Second, pragmatics tends to dictate use of a simple etiological framework. Most other models of smoking development involve numerous variables. Often these variables need to be broken into subsets to make them testable. Certainly, these other models provide little direction for how to break down a comprehensive social influences curriculum into general components. In a study such as Project TNT, it is only pragmatically feasible to test perhaps two or three components in an experimental design. Other models might demand the testing of six or more curricula to provide a complete test of their models. Thus this two-component model of social influence was selected for an important heuristic reason—that of testability of components through an experimental manipulation. Other models can only be tested through use of various statistical modeling approaches, which provide weaker tests than that which can be provided in an experimental analysis.

NOT FORGETTING THE POTENTIAL IMPORTANCE OF TEACHING PHYSICAL CONSEQUENCES IN PREVENTION

Little research has been completed to try to maximize the effectiveness of tobacco use prevention programming oriented toward physical consequences, especially in comparison with the growth of interest in social-influences-oriented research and interventions. Rather, tobacco use prevention researchers have assumed that physical consequences programs are ineffective (McCaul & Glasgow, 1985). This process of research tends to reflect the way that zeitgeists shift. Accidental intervention successes along with a preparedness for conceptual change often lead a research community to a very different shift in research emphasis (Boring, 1957). It remains unclear, however, why previous tobacco use prevention programs oriented toward physical consequences were unsuccessful. There are at least two possible reasons. First, these programs simply may have been *boring* in content or poorly implemented. Second, they may have delivered material that was *irrelevant* to the etiology of tobacco use among adolescents. The next several paragraphs will discuss these two reasons.

Physical Consequences Programs as Boring or Poorly Implemented

Some tobacco use prevention studies have used physical-consequences-oriented programs as placebo programs to compare against comprehensive social influence programs. Placebo programs are introduced in experimental research to control for influences of extratheoretical effects on program outcomes (Kazdin & Wilcoxon, 1976; McGuire, 1969; Shapiro & Morris, 1971). Such program comparisons are advances relative to use of no treatment controls. Extratheoretical effects of a condition can be measured through assessments of students' program success expectancies (Shapiro & Morris, 1971; Sussman, Dent, Brannon, et al., 1989). Johnson (1981) wrote that one of the reasons for the success of the early social influence programs may have been that the control school programs, which were oriented to physical consequences, did not provide equal attention to students. When level of classroom activity, degree of student activation, and quality of instruction were made equivalent, results sometimes did not differ between programs, particularly among males (also see O'Neill, Glasgow, & McCaul, 1983). Only a few smoking prevention researchers have used attention-placebo programs to control for extratheoretical effects such as special attention (e.g., Flay et al., 1988; Schinke & Gilchrist, 1985; Schinke, Gilchrist, Schilling, Snow, & Bobo, 1986).

Unfortunately, even fewer prevention studies have tried to equate subjects' program success expectancies across experimental and placebo conditions. Programs may provide equal time/attention to participants, yet participants may still differ in expectancies for success across conditions due to differences in other extratheoretical variables. For example, Borkovec and Nau (1972) found that ratings of credibility were often lower in attention-placebo than relatively successful therapy groups. Creating parallel conditions, except for theoretically relevant components, allows for a high level of control over program success expectancies across conditions (Kazdin & Wilcoxon, 1976). Using such carefully structured conditions is especially useful in cigarette smoking prevention research, in which the locus of program effects is unclear (Flay, 1985; Flay & Best, 1982; Johnson, 1981; McCaul & Glasgow, 1985). Ultimately, though, equivalent expectancy of conditions must be empirically established.

In an attempt to equate program success expectancies, the Television, School, and Family Smoking Prevention Project (Project TVSFP; Sussman, Dent, Brannon, et al., 1989) designed two programs that differed in content but were similar in procedure (social influences program, long-term physical consequences program). Both programs used role playing as a teaching strategy. In the social influence program, students role-played saying no to tobacco offers, whereas in the physical consequences program, students role-played having tobacco-related diseases such as lung cancer. Fourteen middle schools were randomly assigned to the two programs. As hypothesized, baseline expectancies were found to predict outcome measures even after controlling for baseline smoking intentions, ethnic group, and gender. Second, the equivalence of program expectancies at posttest was tested. Youths held equivalent overall expectancies for success across conditions. Thus program expectancies can be controlled for by equating process of program delivery. A similar process was accomplished in Project TNT (Sussman, Dent, Stacy, Hodgson, et al., 1993; discussed in Chapter 8 of this book), by development of a physical consequences curriculum. As discussed in Chapter 9, the Project TNT physical consequences condition, equated in expectancy for program success with the other conditions, was superior to single-component social influence programs. Thus controlling for expectancy effects may be a main reason that previous physical-consequences-oriented prevention programs were not successful.

Physical Consequences Programs as Irrelevant to Youth

Physical consequences programming may have been irrelevant to youth for four reasons: reliance on long-term consequences material, inadequate instruction of risk of consequences material, inadequate manipulation of fear, or inattention to myths regarding effects of tobacco use among adolescents. Four different possibilities have been researched as ways in which physical consequences program material might be made more relevant to adolescents. One possibility is to teach short-term rather than long-term physical consequences information (e.g., coughing and addiction versus lung cancer). Long-term effects information is unlikely to be accessed by teenagers, most of whom tend not to place much importance on long-term future events. Emphasizing the instruction of relatively short-term physical consequences material, therefore, may be one means of providing youth with information that will lead them to decide against tobacco use. However, in a review of five studies that compared provision of short-term consequences information with long-term consequences information or other material, McCaul and Glasgow (1985) concluded that no study showed provision of immediate consequences information to be superior to provision of long-term effects information. Also, although there was some evidence of an effect of providing any type of consequences information as compared to a standard care (no-treatment) control, placebo effects were not controlled for. Thus provision of health consequences information may be important, but type of information may not be of importance to prevention efforts.

Instruction in the relatively high probability of health risks related to tobacco use must be provided in a way that adolescents can appreciate at a personal level. A second possibility for making physical consequences programs more relevant to youth might be to find an appropriate means to manipulate the presentation of the probability of consequences. Tyler and Cook (1984) hypothesized that when an intervention defines a social or physical condition as a problem and shows in a dramatic and *convincing* way how this problem has affected certain people in the population, *and* when the *frequency of occurrence is high* or the individual *identifies* with the problem, it is possible that people will revise their estimations of the risks involved, both to society and to themselves. Otherwise, individuals tend to underestimate the risks associated with a problem such as tobacco use, at least to themselves (Hansen & Mallotte, 1986; Leventhal, Glynn, & Fleming, 1987; Tyler & Cook, 1984; Weinstein, 1982). Sussman, Dent, Flay, et al. (1989) tested this hypothesis by developing four videos that orthogonally manipulated information about smokeless tobacco use. Specifically, they manipulated convincingness of consequences and probability of consequences in a two-by-two experimental design. They measured personal identification as an individual difference variable, based primarily on previous exposure to use of smokeless tobacco by self or family. The results indicated that probability of consequences more than convincingness of consequences increased personal level of concern about smokeless tobacco use. In addition, the effectiveness of each condition was enhanced by personal identification with smokeless tobacco use. These authors concluded that convincingness of consequences need not influence one's concern toward one's community or oneself. The effects of smokeless tobacco use or other health-related behaviors are fairly well known, and repeating these effects in a dramatic way may be more interesting, or may invoke more sympathy for victims of these consequences, but apparently do not alter one's concerns for self or others in general. Probability of consequences, on the other hand, may be expected to exert a major impact on one's concerns to oneself and to others. People are not likely to want to place themselves or their peers in situations involving high chances of negative consequences. The key to manipulating information on the probability of a consequence perhaps entails presenting it in terms of "relative" rather than "absolute" probability. If a consequence is presented *relative* to nonuse (e.g., the individual is x times as likely to suffer a consequence), the probability of suffering that consequence apparently seems quite high to an audience. On the other hand, the *absolute* probability of suffering that same consequence (e.g., x out of every 1,000 people will suffer the consequence) may seem quite remote. Using relative probability information to convey consequences shows some promise and was made part of the successful Project TNT physical consequences curriculum.

A third possibility for making physical consequences programs more relevant to youth is to manipulate the fear induced by the communication. Although Sussman, Dent, Flay, et al. (1989) did manipulate convincingness/dramatic portrayal of their smokeless tobacco consequences material, no increase in personal level concern was achieved. Perhaps, then, they did not induce fear. Sutton and Eiser (1984) successfully induced fear in a sample of adult smokers in a two-group experimental design by showing or not showing a very frightening physical consequences film that portrayed the last days of a smoker who was dying of lung cancer. This study demonstrated smoking reductions and self-reported cessation in their sample 3 months after viewing the movie, which was predicted directly by induction of fear. Project TNT attempted to achieve this effect in its physical consequences condition by portraying imagery of horrific consequences of use and holding a mock funeral for a youth who died of oral cancer related to smokeless tobacco use.

A fourth possibility for making physical consequences programs more effective is to tie consequences information together as reflecting physical outcomes of different stages of smoking development. By doing so, myths about tobacco use are corrected. For example, first cigarette smoking experiences often are unpleasant physiologically but then become gradually more pleasant (youth stop coughing and stop feeling dizzy or nauseated). Youth may come to learn and believe an illusion that when coughing stops in early smoking experimentation, one is getting *used* to smoking. In prevention programming, they are taught that what is really happening is that their bodily defense systems are giving in, that they are just starting to become addicted to nicotine (Glynn et al., 1985). In an experimental study involving random assignment of classes to conditions, a group receiving a prevention program that corrected this getting-used-to-smoking illusion and other tobacco-use-related myths was compared to an attention control group shown long-term consequences films. The experimental condition achieved a relatively successful preventive effect on levels of smoking beyond trying that held for 18 months postintervention (Hirschman, Leventhal, Fleming, & Glynn, 1987). This smoking developmental correction concept was readily incorporated into the Project TNT physical consequences curriculum.

Sampling, Design, and Tracking Issues

External and internal validity are primary methodological features to be maximized in any prevention program. *Internal validity* refers to the ability to assert that experimental treatments made a difference in a specific instance, whereas *external validity* refers to the generalizability of a finding to other populations (Campbell & Stanley, 1973). To maximize both types of validity in a field study, several basic issues should be considered:

1. Recruitment of schools and sampling of subjects that will provide data representative of the target population
2. Demonstration of random assignment to conditions
3. Examination of the data using appropriate units of analysis while achieving adequate statistical power
4. Collection of accurate data while addressing human-subject consent issues
5. Confounds such as testing and implementer effects, which also need to be addressed
6. Attrition of subjects, which needs to be accounted for
7. Statistical modeling of mediators and moderators, which deserves some discussion as a means of examining statistically why effects are obtained

Project TNT addressed these methodological features, as outlined in the following 10 sections of this chapter.

PROJECT TNT SCHOOL RECRUITMENT

Project TNT used a stratified random selection procedure to select schools for investigation. Blocked by ethnic composition, school size, and rural/urban region, a total of 48 junior high schools (24 rural and 24 urban junior high schools) and 24 high schools (6 rural California, 6 suburban California, 6 rural Illinois, and 6 urban Illinois) were gathered from 29 school districts in southern California and 10 districts in Illinois. In each case, entire districts participated in the project. In order to be included in the study, school personnel agreed to make a 5-year commitment and to have schools randomly assigned to conditions (Craig, Dent, & Sussman, 1988).

The ultimate targets of the proposed interventions and assessments were 7th-grade junior high school students, and senior high school students—the senior high school students being from the 9th, 10th, 11th, and 12th grades. All students were enrolled in public junior high and high schools. Although the study sample was proposed to be simply from "a large and defined" population, an attempt was made to incorporate random sampling techniques in order to approximate samples of more general representativeness.

Students are naturally clustered together in classrooms, schools, and school districts. It was determined that school districts would function as the primary sampling units (PSUs) because school district personnel typically play an important role in the acceptance of study involvement and the long-term adoption of educational programs. They were also selected as PSUs because district-level approval is ultimately necessary in order to freely access individual schools and students.

Recruitment took place in all schools within a sampled district that contained the prevention program target grade (7th). This is typically termed *complete cluster sampling* within the PSU. High schools were selected as those schools that were "fed" by the selected junior high schools in southern California. High schools chosen in Illinois had demographic characteristics similar to those chosen in California.

A complete printed list of all the school district names in southern California, which included the location (county, city, and zipcode) of the superintendent's office and the grade span of schools in the district, was acquired. Next, the "sampling frame" was constructed defining stratification characteristics within which we wanted specific numbers of units (schools).

The first major stratification variable was urban versus rural geographic identification. *Urban* was defined using the U.S. Bureau of the Census's delineation of "urbanized areas," which provides a better separation of urban and rural populations in the vicinity of large cities than Standard Metropolitan Statistical Areas (SMSAs). An urbanized area consists of a central city or cities that, when combined with surrounding closely settled territory (urban fringe), have a population density of at least 1,000 persons per square mile. Typically, urbanized areas cover the built-up area at the core of SMSAs and cover much less area than SMSAs, which, by definition, must be composed of whole counties. *Rural* was defined as any area not defined by the Bureau of the Census as urbanized in 1980 (U.S. Bureau of the Census, 1983). An equal number of schools from the urban and rural strata were sampled in this study.

County was also a stratification variable used in our sampling plan. Using the above definition of urban and rural, together with a distance restriction explained below, we sampled districts from one urban and four rural counties. Each rural county had a varying number of eligible districts, and selection took place within county strata in an attempt to balance the number of districts across counties.

Restrictions

Our sampling frame was further defined by our placing several eligibility restrictions. These were, in order of application:

1. *Grade Span*—Districts that did not span a 7th through 8th grade were eliminated from the sampling frame because they were outside of the study target population. We wanted to sample 48 schools within the junior high school stratum and 12 schools within the high school stratum in southern California. *Junior high school* was defined as any school with 7th- and 8th-grade students, and *high school* was defined as any school with 9th- through 12th-grade students.

2. *Distance*—Districts with schools outside an approximately 150-mile radius or further away from our institute worksite were eliminated due to logistic constraints. This left districts in regions of approximately equal area in the entire largely urbanized counties of Los Angeles and Orange, and parts of the largely rural surrounding counties of Riverside, San Bernardino, Kern, and Ventura. We do not consider this restriction as necessarily biasing the selection process, for the remaining area is quite large and includes school districts with a wide range of characteristics.

3. *Other Ongoing Studies*—Districts in urban Orange County were not considered for our sampling plan but left available for Project SHOUT, another NCI-sponsored project based in San Diego (Elder et al., 1993). Los Angeles County districts involved in other ongoing Institute for Health Promotion and Disease Prevention Research studies (AAPT, SHARP, TVSFP; e.g., Hansen & Graham, 1991) also were not considered eligible for our sample. We do not necessarily view this as overly restrictive to our sampling plan because of the large pool of eligible urban districts (i.e., 61) available in Los Angeles County.

4. *Majority White Ethnicity*—Districts that did not contain a majority of white students were eliminated from the sampling frame. This restriction was applied because of the known higher rates of use of one of the target substances (smokeless tobacco) among this ethnic group. In other words, we oversampled nonethnic minority school districts in order to increase our measurement precision on the behavior of interest. Only those districts with a 50% minimum white composition were chosen.

5. *School Size*—For this calculation, the junior high school target grade was Grade 7. Grade 10 was chosen as the high school target grade because the 10th grade tends to be the largest within most high schools (before students begin to drop out). Districts that contained only extremely small schools (fewer than 50 in the junior high school target grade) and districts with extremely large schools (more than 500 students in the junior high school target grade) were eliminated from the sampling frame because districts with schools of those sizes were atypical. This restriction also eliminated many schools with atypical formats, such as fine arts or continuation high schools, and very large schools, within which implementation of the project would be most difficult.

Procedure

The procedure used by Project TNT to construct lists of school districts that it would attempt to recruit was as follows:

1. We compiled a "complete" unrestricted sampling frame (list) of school districts for each county by marking copies of the printed district list to indicate districts in that county.

2. A computer database containing all California zipcodes and counties was obtained and subset to include only Los Angeles, Ventura, Kern, San Bernardino, and Riverside counties. A (pseudo) random number was computer generated for each zipcode/county entry in the database and attached to the record. The records were then sorted by this random number, and lists were printed for each county. A random sample of zipcodes within counties was achieved by simply choosing in order from the top to the bottom of the randomly ordered zipcode lists.

3. We matched the randomly selected zipcodes in order to the corresponding school districts by searching (by hand) for the entry in the school districts list. Districts that did not contain schools with the desired grade span (included 7th and 8th grades) were eliminated at this point.

4. We defined the districts as either urban or rural by looking up the central office (supervisor's) city classification in the Census Bureau publication *1980 Census of Population and Housing: Geographic Identification Code Scheme* (U.S. Bureau of the Census, 1983).

5. The district office location was looked up in a Thomas Brothers map to determine if it was outside of a 150-mile radius from the city of Pasadena, where the institute was located. If the selected district was outside of the range, it was eliminated at this point.

6. Lists of other schools participating in projects conducted by the Institute for Health Promotion and Disease Prevention Research were checked to see if the selected district was involved in other ongoing projects. The district was eliminated at this point if it contained schools on the other project lists.

7. The CBEDS (California Board of Education Data) archival data was referenced at this point in the selection procedure. District statistics were checked for major white ethnic distribution. Nonmajor (less than 50%) white districts were eliminated at this point. School size statistics were also checked, and if all target schools in the district were either too small (fewer than 50 students in Grade 7), or too large (more than 500 students in Grade 7), the district was eliminated.

8. Districts passing all of the above sampling criteria were listed on a sample selection sheet and given to the project manager for attempted recruitment. The final list divided schools by urban/rural status. The project manager was to randomly select districts from each region in this list until a sufficient sample of schools ($N = 48$ junior high schools) was recruited.

After receiving randomized school district lists, the project manager would contact the school district superintendent and make an appointment to speak with him or her. The project manager then sent a letter to confirm the appointment, met with the appropriate administrative-level person, provided a project overview, explained the project in more detail, and then answered any questions. Routes to participation, reasons for participation, and reasons for nonparticipation are shown in Table 5.1.

All districts acquired were successfully maintained throughout the study. Because involvement with the schools involved a 5-year commitment, Project TNT staff felt that establishing and maintaining a good rapport with each school was imperative. Project TNT found that it is easier to schedule and to do assessments at schools where there is a high level of interest and commitment, and that this can only be developed and maintained through frequent communication. The project manager found it valuable to communicate frequently by telephone or mail (an average of three times per semester). Project TNT kept district contacts and school principals informed and expressed appreciation for their participation in order to strengthen the commitment to work together. For example, before and after each assessment, the project manager sent letters to the district contact person, school principal, and all teachers who had classes that were involved in the studies. Also, holiday greeting cards were sent to help enhance relations with the schools.

STUDENT SAMPLING

Random assignment refers to the process of randomly assigning units to conditions so that (a) any unit has an equal probability of being in any condition, and (b) units so assigned are equivalent or comparable across conditions (Campbell & Stanley, 1973). This was achieved in Project TNT, indicating support for the internal validity of the interventions. Project TNT used two methods of student sampling. In Cohort 1, a complete sample of students from the target grade classes at each of 20 schools was surveyed. This was achieved by use of the active/passive consent protocol

Table 5.1 Project TNT Recruitment Procedure

Routes to School Participation	Number of Districts (of 29 Participating Districts)
Superintendent's and/or district-level approval	10
District's and principals' approval	8
District/board approval—requiring vote	5
District, principals', and 7th/10th-grade teachers' approval	3
Superintendent's, principals', and board's approval	2
District approval, board point of information— no vote required	1

Reasons for Participation	Number of Districts (of 29 Participating Districts)
Interested in being part of research study, wants curriculum and training promised in Year 5	29
No cost to districts or schools and minimal disruption to school functioning	29
Not enough or any drug prevention programs or activities at schools and wants some or more	25
Enhancement of other drug programs (i.e., Here's Looking at You 2000, Quest)	4
Participated in other studies and found it to be a valuable experience	1

Reasons for Nonparticipation	Number of Districts (of 8 Nonparticipating Districts)
Involvement in too many other drug programs and/or activities (overload)	4
Administrative reevaluation and reorganization (unable to make 5-year commitment at this time)	2
Lack of board majority or unanimous vote to approve participation	2

Total number of districts contacted	37
Number of participating districts	29
Number of nonparticipating districts	8
Percentage of districts contacted that participated	78%

described later in this chapter. Actively consented students in Cohort 1 provided confidential identifying information that allowed the linking of data across repeated measurements at an individual level. This cohort provided data in a classic longitudinal fashion where changes in individuals were monitored. Students in Cohort 1 schools who failed to return consent forms were surveyed anonymously. Although data from these students could not be linked at an individual level, they provided information at the school level.

In Cohort 2, a partial sample of three classes of students from each of 28 other schools was surveyed under a strictly anonymous and passive consent procedure. Data from these students provided information at the school level only and could not be linked at an individual level or to individual students. Both cohorts could provide school level data (i.e., smoking prevalence estimates) for longitudinal analysis at the school level (Dent & Sussman, 1990).

The decision to use two different student sampling cohorts, like many other issues in this study, came as a compromise after we considered monetary and informational costs. Anonymous student partial sampling, as in Cohort 2, is all that is strictly necessary for the purposes of program effectiveness evaluation. Estimates of school smoking prevalence and/or other means provide the information needed to determine risk levels for individual schools: that is, whether a school is "high risk" for tobacco use as compared to other schools. This type of sampling eliminates the need and the cost of active consenting and tracking (linkage) of individual students across measurement intervals. However, anonymous sampling (partial or complete) also limits the ability to look at changes in important individual difference variables that may coincide with changes in program outcomes (e.g., risk taking or "high-risk group" membership) at a classic individual level. The ability to conduct these types of auxiliary studies was important. Therefore both types of cohorts were initiated. Anonymous partial sampling is also atypical of prior research designs on tobacco use prevention, and it was feared that the study might not be accepted by the research community unless it had, at least in part, a typical student sampling plan.

EXPERIMENTAL DESIGN

A five-group randomized block design was employed (e.g., Graham, Flay, Johnson, Hansen, & Collins, 1984). Schools were randomly assigned within blocks defined by region (urban, rural), school type (middle school with 6th through 8th grades, junior high school with only 7th through 8th grades), and a composite variable. The composite variable was a linear composite of school size, socioeconomic status (Aid to Family of Dependent Children percentile rank, English as a second language [LEP] percentile rank, median income in zipcode), academic status (California Assessment Program reading, writing, and math percentile ranks), demographic variables (percent white, percent growth of population in zipcode, county name, median age in zipcode), and estimate of tobacco use prevalence (based on school staff estimates and pilot data collected at the school) (Dent, 1989; Dent, Sussman, & Flay, 1993).

A total of 48 junior high schools from 29 southern California school districts were recruited and randomly assigned to participate in one of five conditions. There were eight schools in each of four program conditions, and there were 16 schools in a "standard care" control condition. Students consisted of two cohorts. In Cohort 1, all students from 7th-grade classes at 20 schools were surveyed in an individual-level collection. In Cohort 2, students from 28 other schools were surveyed as repeated cross-sectional partial samples (approximately three classes per school). In each of the four program conditions, 4 schools were urban and 4 were rural; 4 schools were involved in individual-level collection, and the other 4 schools were involved in a repeated cross-sectional collection. Region-by-collection variables were fully crossed. In the control condition, 8 schools were urban and 8 were rural; 4 schools were involved in individual-level collection (half rural/ half urban), and 12 were involved in a repeated cross-sectional collection (half rural/half urban).

In the control condition, students received prevention activities provided directly by their schools. Aside from two lessons in the health education classes—which provided information about tobacco products and long-term consequences—the 16 control schools' activities related to prevention of tobacco use were limited to assemblies that taught values clarification material, long-term physical consequences information, or simple "just say no to drug use" messages (e.g., red ribbon week). None of the control schools provided other programming for tobacco use prevention, although

5 of the 16 control schools did provide at least five lessons of drug use prevention material.

CONSIDERATION OF MULTICOHORT, MULTIYEAR DESIGNS

One possibility that was considered but excluded from the design of Project TNT was the presentation of a multiyear program in which one or more cohorts might receive treatment spread over 2 years (e.g., a combined condition taught to 7th and 8th graders concurrently and then taught to the same students at 8th and 9th grades). Although multicohort, multiyear programs have appeal, a number of problems emerged when we considered them for inclusion in Project TNT. First, costs for adding additional schools to those already receiving the intervention would be greatly increased because the number of schools would at least double. Second, multiyear programs would introduce additional methodological concerns that are not easily resolved. For example, should such a program be repeated in its entirety at the later grade, or should it be split in some way so that the total time of exposure to this multiyear curriculum is equal to that of single-year programs? Third, it was unclear which other grade should be chosen (other than 7th grade). An adjacent age cohort might not command enough justification to replicate the curricula with a doubled N, whereas a much older cohort might be more appropriate for cessation programming. Further, the proportion of students who would actually receive both installments of treatment might be substantially reduced by students changing schools, scheduling irregularities, and so forth. The biases introduced by attrition or disjoint junior/senior high school feeder patterns might render the evaluation of such an approach difficult. Instead, we provided equivalent-length programs to the same age cohort during the same class year. Also, we chose schools with 7th- to 8th-grade transitions to minimize attrition effects at the 1-year follow-up. The issue of multicohort, multiyear programming is interesting and should be pursued. Indeed, others are conducting multiyear programs (e.g., Dr. Art Peterson's tobacco use prevention group in Washington; Boyd & Glover, 1989). However, compared to other concerns addressed by Project TNT (e.g., the main theoretical emphasis being on a test of two major views of the prevention of tobacco use onset and experimentation, statistical power issues), this design possibility was clearly less important and, in the estimation of Project TNT, did not warrant inclusion in this study.

STATISTICAL POWER

Estimating power is a necessary part of any research project, especially large-scale research projects where considerable time and effort are involved (e.g., Rossi, 1990). If there is insufficient power to detect true differences between experimental groups, then erroneous conclusions regarding the lack of potential treatment effectiveness will emerge. In calculating statistical power, there are at least two major issues to consider. The first issue is that of selecting the most appropriate unit of analysis. This has implications for interpretation of degrees of freedom in estimating power. From a methodological point of view, it has been argued (Cook & Campbell, 1979) that the unit of analysis should be the same as the unit of random assignment because that unit is the one most defensibly linked to the concepts of statistical error (Type I and Type II). In many previous research and demonstration projects, it has not been possible to use the school (or other aggregate assignment unit) as a meaningful analysis unit because typically only a few schools were available for experimental and control conditions. This meant that either there were too few units to perform meaningful statistical comparisons or, in those studies with multiple treatment packages per school, that the lack of statistical independence between units was suspect due to between-condition contamination.

In the Project TNT prevention trial, there were a minimum of eight schools per comparison group for the major hypothesis tests, with each school receiving a logically independent treatment package. Thus comparisons of experimental interest permitted Project TNT to perform the study using the school as the unit of analysis (Barcikowski, 1981). Schools are the most appropriate analysis unit for the major tests of experimental hypotheses, but for analyses exploring the mediation of treatment receptivity by those variables not experimentally balanced or controlled, other levels must be used as the unit of analysis. Classrooms may be more appropriate units in analysis involving treatment implementation and process evaluations if there is considerable intraschool variability among classrooms. For those analyses involving individual differences variables, the individual is clearly the most appropriate unit of analysis. At each level of disaggregation (classroom within school, individual within classroom), Project TNT's sampling design included a sufficient number of subunits so that gains in degrees of freedom, and hence in statistical power, adequately offset any additional variability in the standard errors of the statistical tests performed within those units. Project TNT did not consider for purposes of power calculation, at the time of determining the experimental design, use of mixed-model random regression models for clustered data, which adjust for dependence among included observations grouped into classrooms and schools (Burnstein, 1980; Donner, 1982, 1985; Hedeker, Gibbons, & Flay, 1994). Future research might consider this possibility to facilitate a more liberal power calculation (Koepke & Flay, 1989).

A second issue to be considered when calculating statistical power for an experimental test is that the information needed to determine the power (i.e., the true mean difference induced by the treatment and the population standard deviation) is seldom known in advance, but must be estimated. If these estimates are reasonably accurate, then good decisions can be made about the size of the effect that can be detected. However, if these estimates are inaccurate, in some cases even by a relatively small amount, then what initially appeared to be a good chance of detecting a true program effect (e.g., power about .90) may turn out to be closer to a 50/50 chance of finding an effect. Thus in determining power the project was guided by several statistically conservative principles (Cohen, 1977; Cohen & Cohen, 1979).

First, the power analysis was aimed at the primary hypotheses of the study (condition comparisons) because effect size estimates are likely to be the most accurate for these. Although it is numerically possible to compute the power of a very complicated analysis, power analysis for a simpler analysis is likely to be more accurate. Second, calculations were not point estimates, but examined expected power over a range of true differences between groups centered on our "best guess" estimates of treatment effects. Third, given that testing of primary hypotheses was the major purpose of the experiment, these main effects would have a rather overwhelming chance of being detected (power greater than .80). In this way, the tests of secondary hypotheses that might emerge through the exploration of the numerous program mediators would have at least some chance of detecting true effects. And finally, power was calculated using the primary (and appropriate) unit of analysis planned for the actual analysis of the data. Because schools were used in the analysis of primary treatment comparisons, those units determined the degrees of freedom in the power calculations. Power for the major planned comparisons was computed for several different effect sizes based on regional smokeless tobacco prevalence data presented by Boyd and Associates (1987).

Certain assumptions were made regarding anticipated effects in the prevention component of Project TNT. One was that, based on previous interventions of this type, Project TNT expected to reduce the onset of smokeless tobacco by as much as 50% in the single-strategy programs. In the combined-strategy program, an additional 25% reduction in use was assumed possible due to the broader manipulation. The large effect ($d = .8$) was based on these expected maximum effect sizes. The medium ($d = .4$) and small ($d = .2$) effect sizes coincided with those defined by Cohen (1977). It was further assumed that any increase in use would be linear over the 24-month assessment period (between the beginning of the 7th to the 9th grade), and that program effects would be maintained over the 2-year follow-up interval. At the early assessments, the chances of detecting a large-sized effect were all reasonably good, the smallest power value being .75 in the comparison contrasting the effectiveness of any two single-strategy programs. By the one-year follow-up, all comparisons had power greater than .80 for a true medium-sized effect. At the 2-year follow-up, even small effects had a reasonable chance of being detected (minimum power = .82), assuming than the program effects were maintained to that point. The overall main effect comparison (all programs versus either control) had power over .88 to detect even small, early effects. From these data, it was concluded that the school sample size was approximately the right size to provide acceptable statistical power.

CONSENT PROCEDURES

There are two types of parallel consent procedures (Dent, Galaif, et al., 1993; Severson & Ary, 1983). An active consent procedure is one in which subjects are asked to have their parents sign and return the consent letter providing written permission or refusal for participation in the program or any part of the testing. For those parents who do not sign a form, a human subjects review committee can approve a verbal consent through telephone contact. In a passive consent procedure, parents are informed that students from whom active verbal dissent has not been obtained will be considered to have been provided consent from parents for engagement in the collection procedure.

Over the last several years, an increasing trend has been to allow a passive consent procedure only for collection of anonymous data. In an anonymous data collection protocol, student surveys are identified by a number only. Only the classroom and school are noted, making linkage of the survey response to individual names impossible. This type of collection is useful for school-level or classroom-level analyses only. Maximizing consent returns has been an ongoing concern in school-based prevention research because those who do not return consents tend to have children who are more likely to be tobacco users (see Dent, Galaif, et al., 1993; Severson & Ary, 1983). Further, such parents apparently present an apathetic attitude toward their children, or at least spend less time with their children (Dent, Galaif, et al., 1993; Richardson et al., 1989).

The difficulty in maximizing consent return rates sometimes occurs when collecting confidential, individual-level data, which requires active consent. A consent rate of at least 70% is desired to obtain a reasonable sample size for longitudinal research, but active consent is quite difficult to achieve relative to passive consent. To obtain a 70% active consent response, Project TNT tested various means of sending information home to parents and obtaining written approval or disapproval from them. The data collection team tested two means of completing this procedure: (a) sending project information home along with other packets normally sent by the school (i.e., school information packets or quality evaluation packets); and (b) distributing materials, including consent forms, in the classroom where they would be measured. The consents were handed out either by a TNT staff member following a brief presentation or by an informed teacher, as close to the assessment date as possible to reduce the probability of consents getting lost or being forgotten. The first protocol resulted in a consent return rate of approximately 50%, whereas the classroom distribution protocol resulted in a return of approximately 62%. In some cases the consents were redistributed by the teacher to increase the return rate. Explained below are the methods of redistribution.

Active Consent Redistribution

When possible the redistribution was accomplished by the teacher whose classroom time would be used for collection. Every effort was made to simplify what was required by school staff.

One method of redistribution was to give every student a new consent. A second was for Project TNT staff to obtain the rosters of classes to be used for collection and to determine which students had not yet been given consent. The school was then given additional consents and a list of students needing consent. This approach was taken further in a third method of actually writing the students' names on the consent form, which simplified distribution for the teacher. This method proved to be the most effective.

A meeting was held with either a school consent contact person (assigned to us by the school principal) or the teachers to explain our objectives and request their assistance. Specific dates for distribution and collection of consents were set at that time. Again, the best results occurred when the teachers were informed and involved.

Generally teachers and school staff made every effort to get the consents returned. For example, in one school, students were given the incentive of a school reward for returning the consent. In most schools, the teachers simply increased their effort to get a parental response. Even with their support, and active consent redistribution, the overall return rate was only 64%. Further methods were designed to increase return.

Verbal Active Consent

Our project staff proposed an active verbal consenting procedure to the University of Southern California Research Committee (Institutional Review Board), which was approved. Data collection staff contacted the parents or guardians directly by phone. The California State Education Codes 49076 and 76243 provide for the release of student directory information from school districts to agencies involved in research.

The verbal consent procedure was used in schools where phone numbers were available. Data collection staff were scheduled to call between 4:00 p.m. and 8:30 p.m., with occasional calls being made during the daytime. Some weekend calls were made at schools requiring more calling time, but our experience and that of other projects indicated that weekends were poor times to call. Early evening was the best time to reach the largest number of parents. On the average, a caller was able to complete 10 calls per hour. Because 27% of the sample were Hispanic students, bilingual callers were employed.

Callers followed a strict protocol and script when contacting a parent. Parents were told that consent materials had been sent home and were asked if they had received them or were familiar with the project. The project was explained in detail to parents who had not been informed, and callers offered to mail duplicate consent forms directly to their homes. Parents were then asked to verbally consent or decline.

The information documented for each call was (a) name of the person giving consent, (b) his or her relationship to the student, (c) time and day of the call, (d) the name and extension of the caller, and (e) if it was a verbal consent or a verbal decline. Evidence of these calls also was backed up by phone bills. When consent forms were sent to the homes, parents were asked to either return them to the schools or forward them directly to the institute in enclosed self-addressed, stamped envelopes. The rate of parental approval brought the active consent rate up to 75% overall. The no-contact rate across all schools was 14%.

Passive Consent Distribution

With all active consent avenues exhausted, the overall consent rate was 75%. It was then decided that a passive consent should be distributed to all students who had not received consent 1 to 2 weeks before the collection date. These students would participate in an anonymous survey on collection day if a parental decline was not returned. In schools where student addresses were available, the passive consents were mailed home via first-class mail one week prior to the date of collection. In districts where this information was not available, the teachers were asked to distribute passive consents to students who had not received consent one week before collection. Usually students' names were prewritten on the consent, and the teachers were provided with a list of students still needing consent. This procedure increased the overall participation rate an average of approximately 7%, reaching an overall 82% participation rate. In our subsequent data collection, parents were informed in *one* letter that if we did not receive active consent from them, we would assume passive consent for an anonymous collection (unless we received active dissent from the parent).

At passive-consent-only schools, which used a blanket passive consent distribution, absentee rate was 10%, and student or parent dissent was approximately 5% (85% participation). Thus the passive consent participation rate generally was 10% higher than the active-consent-only rate.[1]

EFFECTS OF REPEATED TESTING
ON STUDENT REPORTS

Another methodological issue that was raised in the project was that of short-term repeated testing of students using the same measurement instrument. In the longitudinal study, we planned to repeat measurement of students at an immediate pretest, immediate posttest, one-year follow-up, and 2-year follow-up to evaluate the effectiveness of the interventions. The impact of repeated testing at one-year intervals is of little concern relative to other factors operating over that interval (i.e., sample attrition, intervention "fading"). However, the issue of short-term repeated testing was of concern in this project. This issue arose from logistic as well as methodological concerns over immediate pre- and posttesting around the 2-week project intervention period. The issue was whether to test immediately before the intervention period, immediately after intervention, or at both times.

Given adequate randomization of experimental units (i.e., statistical pretest equivalence), posttest-only designs yield treatment effect information identical to that of pretest-posttest designs. However, it is generally considered that repeated testing (i.e, pretest-posttest) designs are stronger than single-measurement-point designs (i.e, posttest only) because they afford the ability to examine treatment effects between groups even when randomization is absent or fails (Campbell & Stanley, 1973). With this in mind, testing at both pre- and postintervention was warranted, especially for evaluating short-term (i.e., knowledge or intention) intervention effects. However, there are costs and benefits to repeated testing. One cost is the obvious increase in monetary and logistical cost—it takes nearly twice (but not quite) the time and resources to have two measurements as it does one. The question of whether any additional information is obtained with repeated testing, given the probability of adequate randomization, needs to be considered.

Another concern with repeated testing is that of subject reactivity. Subjects may respond to the repeated measurement burden by failing to complete the survey or by responding in atypical ways. Alternatively, by repeatedly taking the survey (or "test" as students may perceive it), the issues and attitudes addressed in the survey may also become more salient, resulting in a seeking out of or hyperattentiveness to the issues.

Because there was some initial concern over the adequacy of the randomization procedure to yield strictly equivalent treatment groups, and because of the scope of the project (i.e., it could barely afford the redundancy, but could not afford to not confirm pretest comparability empirically), a compromise was initiated. The compromise involved introducing the pretest as an additional design factor (administer/not administer), to be crossed and balanced over the existing design factors in a Solomon four-group design (Campbell & Stanley, 1973).

In a Solomon four-group design, one evaluates testing effects by randomly assigning units along two crossed factors: treatment versus control and pretested versus not pretested. By engaging in this design, one can assess the effect of pretesting on students' responses (main effects), which relates to external validity, and assess the impact of pretesting on estimates of treatment effects (interactions), which relates to the internal validity of the experiment. In Project TNT, we actually had four treatment groups and a control group, and pretesting was balanced over all these groups. For the purposes of presentation, we collapsed across the treatment groups.

Analysis was conducted using testing and treatment, and their interaction, as factors using analysis of covariance (ANCOVA). Urban/rural status and the assignment blocking variable were included in all models as covariates. Outcomes examined included the following: the number of items completed; whether subjects lived with both parents; self-report of trial and current use of tobacco and alcohol; social desirability and classroom climate scales; personality scales of risk taking, self-esteem, stress, loneliness, assertiveness, health lifestyle, and future-past time orientation; social influence scales of peer tobacco use, peer approval of tobacco use, prevalence estimates of adolescent tobacco use, peer bonding, and family conflict; and knowledge scales for the three types of curriculum content being presented. We wanted to inflate our ability to find a difference as a means of being cautious regarding the possibility of the operation of testing effects. Thus an individual level of analysis was used. Sample size on any comparison was over 3,000, yielding very sensitive assessment of any potential testing effects.

Results indicated that, overall, short-term repeated testing did not interfere with estimation of treatment effects, nor did it prompt student reactivity. Not one treatment-by-testing interaction effect was found in the analysis, indicating that, in the sample, the internal validity of the experiment was not jeopardized. Project TNT also found no main effect for pretesting on any of the personality or social scales, on the demographic items or social desirability scales, or on reports of tobacco and alcohol use. These results indicate that external validity of the experiment generally was not affected by pretesting. Two differences in pretested groups did emerge. Pretested students completed more items than nonpretested students (144 versus 129 items), and pretested students scored 1% to 2% better on the knowledge scales. As mentioned, neither of these differences interacted with treatment. This result indicated that there is a small amount of information seeking and/or "priming" that occurs with repeated testing. Also, repeated testing yields a small practice effect on our survey, allowing completion of nearly 10% more items.

HEALTH EDUCATOR EFFECTS

A good health educator goes a long way in motivating a preventive effort, regardless of curriculum content. Good health educators tend to be adaptive to different classroom situations, are highly self-monitoring, are considerate of student personalities, are enthusiastic (not burned out), believe in the material they are teaching (are honest), are socially skilled, are well prepared to teach the material and know how to facilitate student participation, use effective classroom management strategies to maximize learning time, teach material quickly but in small steps, tailor material to the classroom, and permit positive interactions with students while maintaining a professional demeanor (Brophy, 1986; Clarke, MacPherson, Holmes, & Jones, 1986; Cleary & Gobble, 1990; Eiseman, Robinson, & Zapata, 1984; Larkin, 1987; Rohrbach, Graham, & Hansen, 1993; Sobol et al., 1989; Young, Elder, Green, de Moor, & Wildey, 1988). Because health educators vary in these qualities and hence differ in the information they are able to provide to students, some means of controlling for difference in quality of health educator performance are needed. There are at least three means to control for health educator performance. First, health educators could be trained to a high level (or criterion) of overall performance. This goal was attempted in Project TNT. Health educators in the project were provided with 2 weeks of training in the four curricula; training involved one-on-one instruction with a trained health educator and use of a detailed health educator's manual. Next, health educators observed the delivery of a full curriculum across multiple classrooms before actually delivering the curriculum themselves. (In fact, four of the eight core health educators were cowriters of at least one of the curricula). However, many projects cannot afford this amount of effort, and even extensive training does not guarantee equivalent delivery across conditions. A second means to control for differential performance is through use of a matching procedure of some type. Simply matching health educators on some overall performance score is one means of controlling for quality of delivery if different health educators teach different program conditions. However, although this is not investigated or currently supported by available literature, different health educators might be differentially effective with different classes or different curricula, such that matching only a few health educators across conditions would not accomplish equivalent delivery of programming. Thus a third means, involving counterbalancing of health educators, may be the best choice (given that all educators are highly trained). In Project TNT, each of seven health educators taught all four curricula (normative social influence oriented, informational social influence oriented, physical consequences oriented, and combined) at least two times, and a total of nine taught all curricula at least once. By rotating health educators through all conditions, we controlled for most potential health education effects. This form of control was suggested by Paul (1966).

ATTRITION AND TRACKING ISSUES

Internal validity refers to the ability to interpret a manipulation, whereas *external validity* refers to generalization. Study attrition or loss of experimental units from the original sample often is cited as a threat to validity. Attrition is related to validity in a number of ways (Hansen, Collins, Malotte, Johnson, & Fielding, 1985). Treatment-by-attrition interactions threaten internal validity, whereas loss of subjects limits generalizability of a study (to those subjects who remain in the study).

Statistical modeling of attrition is one way in which one can infer program outcomes, given that certain populations have left the study (particularly those at higher risk, e.g. Dent, 1988). Intensive tracking of target groups also can be entertained. In Project TNT, subject attrition was dealt with in two distinct ways, which followed generally from the two student sampling cohort designs. In the individual-level cohort (Cohort 1), Project TNT attempted to avoid attrition by intensifying resources to "capture" respondents. In the school-level cohort (Cohort 2), statistical adjustment and sampling procedures were relied upon to account for naturally occurring changes in school composition.

For Cohort 1 schools, the notion of an "intensively tracked" subcohort was introduced. The reasoning behind this subcohort was as follows. There were approximately 3,500 students in the initial Cohort 1. A high follow-up rate was necessary to increase the validity of the study. Obtaining a high proportion of the cohort at follow-up was going to require a great deal of resources (tracking and mailing, phone, or school-assisted measurements). It is fairly well documented that students who stay in the same schools exhibit characteristics that place them less at risk for tobacco use than those who do not (i.e, those that we have to track). It is also fairly well understood that those students who are "easy" to find (in schools or otherwise) are at lower risk than those who are harder to track (Dent, Galaif, et al., 1993; Severson & Ary, 1983).

If the high percentage of follow-up was calculated strictly on the total sample size, a significant amount of resources would be expended to capture a possibly low-risk population. Project staff therefore identified a priori those students who were considered to be at high and low risk of tobacco use based on their initial testing. Subcohorts with equal numbers of high- and low-risk individuals at each school were then constructed. Risk was defined on the crossing of two factors: whether the individual had tried tobacco, and whether he or she scored above or below the median score on a curriculum knowledge index (assessed at immediate posttest). Approximately 80 subjects from each school (20 in each high-low combination) were identified. These 1,600 students then became the base for student tracking efforts, assuring an adequate sample of high-risk individuals.

Cohort 1 schools were "swept" with complete measurement of the target grade. Some effort was made to measure no-shows in Cohort 1, including use of absentee packets or home telephone interviews. Due to cost considerations, exhaustive attempts to reach all individuals in Cohort 1 were not made; extensive tracking efforts were then applied to the intensive subgroup of Cohort 1 students not captured in the sweep. Cohort 2 schools measured students anonymously in three randomly composed classrooms. Both cohorts were asked to report on the survey the name of the school they had attended in the prior year. This information gave us a means of assessing the rate of student turnover in each school, regardless of measurement cohort. The average turnover rate was 7%. As summarized by Graham and Donaldson (1993), attrition can be controlled statistically by modeling of the mechanisms causing attrition. At the school level, the mechanism for attrition *is* turnover, and that variable can serve as an adjustment variable in models of treatment effects. One can apply a similar strategy to the individual cohort (Heckman, 1979) by obtaining an estimate of the probability of dropping out of the study for each individual. We accomplished this goal by using a multivariate logistic regression analysis to predict the binary follow-up status variable. Project TNT found that attrition at one-year follow-up among the individual-level cohort was 20.1% of the original sample, but it was not predicted by treatment condition, any of the personality, social, or knowledge scales, or tobacco use in the multivariate models. Attrition at the one-year follow-up was related to living in an urban area, being nonwhite, living with one parent, and having tried alcohol. Study attrition in Cohort 1 at the 2-year follow-up (high school transition year) was 48.5%. The multivariate logistic regression models showed that we lost uniformly more subjects in all treatment conditions relative to control subjects. Attrition continued to be related to being nonwhite, early alcohol use, and living with single parents, and continued to be unrelated to personality, social, or knowledge scales. The model also showed better 2-year follow-up of those who *had* tried tobacco in 7th grade, probably due to intensive cohort tracking. The results from this investigation indicated that it was necessary to control statistically for study attrition, especially in the 2-year follow-up outcome analysis.

ANALYSIS OF MEDIATION AND MODERATION

Outcomes are modeled in terms of both individual and cluster (grouping) variables. Random regression models have been developed for both continuous (Bock, 1983) and dichotomous (Gibbins & Bock, 1987) single and repeated measurements. The general model can be expressed as follows:

$$Y_{ijkt} = \mu_t + \alpha_{it} + \beta X_{ijkt} + \gamma_{jt} + \varepsilon_{ijkt}$$

where μ = the control (population) grand mean, α = the effect due to treatment i, β = the set of regression coefficients for measure X, γ = the random effect due to school j, ε = the random effect due to subject k (error), i = treatment group index, j = school index, k = subject index, and t = time of measurement.

In our design, the treatment manipulations are constructed with additive components: that is, α_1 = nc, α_2 = ic, α_3 = pc, and $\alpha_4 = \alpha_1 + \alpha_2 + \alpha_3$ = cc, where nc = normative social influence component, ic = informational social influence component, pc = physical consequences component, and cc = combined condition.

The main trial manipulation provided an overall test of the relative effectiveness of the different types of social-influences-oriented and physical-consequences-oriented components. Several alternative etiological concepts could be tested for more specification regarding the mechanisms of effects within components using individual difference measures (i.e., susceptibility to social influences, self-esteem, risk taking, other problem behaviors, expectancies of positive and negative consequences). Individual difference variables may either mediate or moderate treatment effects. Mediator effects generally are considered more specific definitions of mechanisms of action (i.e., to mediate an effect of some treatment; Baron & Kenny, 1986; Lubinski & Humphreys, 1990). Alternatively, moderator effects define different levels of treatment impact independent of the values of X, but do not define the general component (e.g., gender).

The finding of a significant indirect effect of treatment through these measures, after controlling for earlier use, would support a hypothesis concerning the role of mediating influences subsumed by the general component label (e.g., normative social influence). Indirect effects in our models are defined as in MacKinnon et al. (1991) as follows. An indirect effect of X is indicated if

$$\alpha_i - (\beta\alpha \times \beta X) > 0$$

where α, β, i, and X are defined as above. Similarly, we can test for moderator effects of individual differences variables on the impact of the treatment using the interaction terms in our general models by defining the product term $\pi\alpha X$ in

$$Y_{ijkt} = \mu + \alpha_{it} + \beta X_{ijkt} + \gamma_{jt} + \pi\alpha X_{ijkt} + \varepsilon_{ijkt}$$

where X and α are defined as above and π is the regression coefficient for the product. Then a moderator effect of X is indicated if $\pi > 0$.

Discriminant Validity of Prevention Program Components and Plans for Statistical Mediation Analysis

In Project TNT, very distinct curricula have been created (see Chapter 8), and the different curricula show discriminant validity on knowledge item manipulation checks (see Chapter 9; see also Sussman, Dent, Stacy, Hodgson, et al., 1993). The evidence for discriminant validity of learning effects on items that uniquely represent the different treatments suggests that the a priori development of program components was successful. In a true experimental design, such as was the primary aspect of our study, a comparison of program-specific knowledge is a reasonable means to argue that each treatment manipulated distinct concepts as planned.

This type of manipulation check has a much longer history of use in interventions than more recent attempts at statistical tests of mediation (MacKinnon et al., 1991), applying the work of Sobel (1982). In recent statistical mediational analyses, successful drug use prevention programs have not been mediated by more than one or two foci of the intervention. In part, this lack of mediation is due to limitations placed on such an analysis by selection of questionnaire items. For example, such tests are limited by the contents of available mediator measures. Another potential problem in using mediators based on questionnaire measures of psychosocial processes is that mediational effects from such data are usually attenuated due to measurement error (Baron & Kenny, 1986; Judd & Kenny, 1981); although structural modeling techniques can help reduce the likelihood of attenuation, these strategies are not appropriate for our primary analyses, which have been completed at a school unit of analysis. Despite some potential problems in statistical tests of mediation, these tests are worth attempting in evaluation research, are worthy of continued development (e.g., Dwyer, 1983; MacKinnon & Dwyer, 1993), and represent a necessary next step in prevention research (McCaul & Glasgow, 1985).

NOTE

1. Some of this material was contributed by Ms. Custer-Smith (see Custer, Gildea, & Liverman, 1989).

SIX

Alternative Methods of Assessment of Tobacco-Use-Related Variables

The school is a social context where adolescents receive many normative and informational cues from their peers regarding tobacco use behavior (Sussman, 1989). Social information diffuses rapidly in schools as youth move from class to class throughout the day (Flay & Best, 1982). Consequently interschool variability on a variety of social variables is much greater than intraschool variability. Discrete differences in tobacco use acceptability, policy enforcement, prevention program receptivity, and proportion of users exist across schools (Brannon et al., 1989; Dent, Sussman, & Flay, 1993; Pentz, Brannon, et al., 1989).

Schools are considered the primary unit of assignment and level of analysis in school-based prevention research (Dent, Sussman, & Flay, 1993; Graham, Flay, Johnson, Hansen, & Collins, 1984; also recall the last chapter). Prevention researchers need measures of the degree of risk for adolescent tobacco use posed by the school environment that provide an economic means for utilizing randomized block designs.

Not surprisingly, one's own prior use and tobacco use by peers are among the strongest predictors of future tobacco use behavior. Thus the most direct and obvious measure of the degree of risk posed by the school environment for tobacco use among adolescents is assessment of tobacco use obtained through student self-reports in interviews or multiple-choice questionnaire formats (e.g., Graham, Flay, Johnson, Hansen, & Collins, 1984; Pechacek, Fox, Murray, & Luepker, 1984). These methods involve collecting tobacco use information at the individual level and then averaging the information across individuals to provide the school-level estimate. The interview method is relatively time consuming to administer; whereas self-report questionnaires allow access to large numbers of adolescents, are easy to code, and generally are considered to be an objective assessment (Newman & Gillies, 1984). However, there are some limitations to this latter approach: (a) respondents must choose from a fixed set of choices, (b) provisions generally are not made for unexpected outcomes, and (c) respondents are assumed to possess a certain level of literacy (Newman & Gillies, 1984). Also, though providing a good estimation of school-level use, self-report measures take precious time to collect and analyze, may be perceived as intrusive by some students, and may elicit a test reactivity confound in some prevention trials (although this was not found to be the case in Project TNT, other than a small priming effect; see Chapter 5). Of additional practical difficulty, the cost of data collection is quite expensive. Collection, entry, and basic analysis for a typical grade at a California junior high school ($N = 200$) would take 4 days and costs approximately $1,000 (in 1990) without biochemical data collection. Because of the high cost and other potential difficulties produced by the collection of individual-level data, it would be useful to investigate other methods of collecting information about student tobacco use at the school level. In addition, alternative, corroborative measures enable tobacco use to be more accurately measured. Development of reliable and valid self-report measures is established primarily through use of biochemical validation and the use of proxy measures, including archival data. Several such developments have occurred in the tobacco use prevention field to validate tobacco use self-report measures, as reported below.

First, data from a carefully completed student interview study will be presented. Much theoretical richness is derived from such a study even though it is costly to conduct. Afterwards, we present several alternative methods of assessing student tobacco use or tobacco-related theoretical constructs. These methods are biochemical

validation, school personnel interviews, refuse analysis, naturalistic observation, archival data, and store personnel interviews.

STUDENT INTERVIEWS

The structured interview has been used increasingly in cigarette
smoking research, both regarding cessation (e.g., Shiffman, 1982, 1984)
and prevention (Friedman et al., 1985). These research efforts were
made in response to the fact that almost no data are available on the
precise high-risk situations teenagers face (Friedman et al., 1985),
particularly with respect to smokeless tobacco use (Hahn et al., 1990).

Friedman et al. (1985) used an open-ended interview to elicit
information from 157 adolescents about their first three smoking
situations. They found that smoking usually began in group settings
with friends of the same sex and that often another peer was also
smoking for the first time. Students were categorized as nonusers
(those who had never experimented with cigarettes), minimal experimenters (those who had experimented with cigarettes between one
and nine times), and persistent experimenters (those who had experimented with cigarettes 10 or more times). Persistent experimenters
were exposed to the most influences to smoke. In addition, those who
continued smoking reported more pleasant emotional and physiological reactions to their early smoking experiences. In an effort to
replicate their study precisely, Hahn et al. (1990) used the same
tobacco use categories applied by Friedman et al. (1985), as reported
above. However, this latter study differed from theirs because it (a)
asked questions regarding smokeless tobacco as well as cigarettes;
(b) probed into thoughts and feelings just prior to, during, and after
the first and last tobacco use experiences; and (c) asked analogous
questions of nonusers regarding their first and last observations of
use by significant others (see Hahn et al., 1990 for more details).

Project TNT Student Interview Study

Single classrooms from each of four urban junior high schools,
six rural junior high schools, three urban high schools, and three

rural high schools in the southern California area were selected. These 16 schools were randomly selected from a pool of 64 schools participating in a larger study. The 64 schools were randomly identified in a five-county area in and around Los Angeles. Seventh graders were interviewed in the junior high schools, and 10th graders were interviewed in the high schools.

Of the 320 students who participated in the interview, 161 (50.3%) were females, and 60% of the students were 7th graders. In the full sample, use category frequencies were: 103 minimal cigarette experimenters, 65 persistent cigarette experimenters, 43 minimal smokeless tobacco experimenters, 20 persistent smokeless tobacco experimenters, and 140 nonusers.

The primary instruments were a series of structured, open-ended, individual interviews designed to elicit details about the student's first experience with a tobacco product and the student's last experience with a tobacco product. A General Student Interview was administered to all of the students and included items on demographics, knowledge of tobacco laws, knowledge of health warning labels, and tobacco use status of the individual. If a student had experience with cigarettes or smokeless tobacco or both, the student was given corresponding interviews in which these experiences were explored in detail. Students were asked to describe the situation, their thoughts and feelings, other people present, the time and place of the occurrence, other activities occurring simultaneously, pressure exerted by the group, reasons for use, subjective reactions to the tobacco, intentions to use in the future, and thoughts about cessation of use.

Results and Discussion

Many of the cigarette experimentation results of this research were consistent with the results of Friedman et al. (1985). Typically, as was found by the Friedman group, cigarette experimentation took place in same-sex peer and sibling groups. Most experimentation took place in small groups, and usually in the afternoon. The majority of these groups consisted of close friends. Often youth were prompted to use by suggestions from others in the group. Most use occurred at home, at school, or at friends' houses.

The current research did not replicate the findings of Friedman et al. (1985) regarding offers to use. They had found that persistent experimenters received more suggestions from the group to use tobacco than those at lower levels of use. In our study, no evidence was found that the adolescents in the minimal experimentation group and the persistent experimentation group experienced different levels of social encouragement.

In an extension of the previous study, Project TNT found that smokeless tobacco use situations appeared to be similar to cigarette-use situations in that adolescent tobacco experimenters (a) typically experimented in small, same-sex groups; (b) often experimented at home and at friends' houses; (c) often cited curiosity as the reason for finally trying the tobacco; and (d) often received suggestions from others in the group to try tobacco, as well as receiving offers of tobacco from others (i.e., 65% of all students interviewed who had experimented with tobacco products reported receiving such offers). In addition, those who progressed to higher levels of use reported fewer negative physiological reactions and relatively pleasant first-trial experiences. The smokeless tobacco use situations investigated differed from the cigarette experimentation situations reported in that smokeless tobacco experimenters (a) were older when they first tried the product, (b) used more often when playing or watching a sport, (c) were more likely to have asked for the tobacco, (d) did not feel addicted to the tobacco, and (e) were less concerned with a negative reaction from parents.

Nonusers lived in tobacco-using households roughly as often as users. They often described observations of a parent or relative using. Why then did these students abstain from tobacco use? The most often cited reason among nonusers for not experimenting with tobacco was fear of physical consequences. This is interesting in light of the recent belief that prevention curricula that rely on information about physical consequences and fear are ineffective (Flay, 1985; Thompson, 1978). It may be wise to keep the information and fear components in the more state-of-the-art social-influences prevention programs with an emphasis on making the physical consequences more personally relevant to the students (recall the last section of Chapter 4). The majority of the nonusers reported feeling pride in their decisions not to smoke. This may indicate a role of a high self-esteem in preventing tobacco use onset.

BIOCHEMICAL VALIDATION

Researchers have validated students' self-reports by objective physiologic measures. Three biochemical validation methods that have been employed include exhaled carbon monoxide (CO) measurement, saliva thiocyanate (SCN) measurement, and saliva cotinine measurement, with varying reliability.

Carbon monoxide is the largest single component in inhaled cigarette smoke. Expired air CO samples can be analyzed immediately upon collection. Nonsmokers typically have CO readings lower than 10 ppm, and this has become the generally agreed-upon cutoff point to distinguish smokers from nonsmokers. Self-reports of the amount smoked and CO readings are correlated about .48 in adults (Vogt, Selvin, Widdowson, & Hulley, 1977), and CO cannot be selectively removed by cigarette filters (Wynder & Hoffman, 1979). Problems include a relatively short half-life (3-5 hours), and elevated readings from children of smoking households, making it difficult to identify nondaily smokers (Glynn, Gruder, & Jegerski, 1986).

Thiocyanates are found in body fluids, partly as a result of detoxification of hydrogen cyanide in cigarette smoke (Luepker et al., 1981). SCN levels in adults are related to the level of cigarette smoking (Gillies, Wilcox, Coates, Krismundsdottir, & Reid, 1982), and have a half-life of 10 to 14 days (Luepker et al., 1981). The rate of false positives is low, at a cutoff point of ≥ 100 ng/ml; however, unless 10 cigarettes have been smoked in the last 24 hours, this level cannot be reached. As a result, experimental smokers go undetected (Luepker et al., 1981). SCN levels can be inflated by cyanogenic foods such as cabbage (Glynn et al., 1986) and can be influenced by factors that change intercellular fluid volume (e.g., diuresis) (Pechacek et al., 1984).

The measurement of cotinine, a major metabolite of nicotine, is a more precise measure of nicotine intake and has a half-life of 30 hours (McMorrow & Fox, 1983). Salivary cotinine is a reliable alternative to plasma cotinine for validation of smoking status and for following changes in smoking behavior over time (Haley, Axelrod, & Tilton, 1983). Smokeless tobacco users can readily be identified by elevated cotinine levels (Gritz et al., 1981). However, this measure is about five times as expensive as SCN analysis.

Collection and analysis of biologic samples, especially in large-scale research projects, is time consuming, problematic, and expensive (Hansen, Mallotte & Fielding, 1985). The idea of a "bogus pipeline" paradigm, in which subjects are convinced that their self-reports will be validated by objective, physiologic measures that are in fact bogus, was introduced by Jones and Sigall (1971), who recommended "unrestricted" adaptation of the procedure. It has been tested experimentally to encourage adolescents to self-report smoking behavior more accurately. Increased reporting has been assumed to be synonymous with more valid reporting (Campanelli, Dielman, & Shope, 1987). Early research resulted in increased self-reporting; however, later research has placed the bogus pipeline procedure under question.

Evans, Hansen, and Mittelmark (1977) applied the bogus pipeline technique to adolescent smoking behavior. Before completing a questionnaire, the subjects were shown a 3-minute color videotape depicting the detectability of nicotine in saliva samples and were asked to provide a saliva sample. The control group completed the questionnaire only. Confidentiality was also assured. Twice as many subjects reported smoking when data were collected using the bogus pipeline procedure.

These results have been generally supported by Luepker et al. (1981), who found increased self-reporting among 7th-grade smokers, but not experimenters, when the bogus pipeline procedure was employed. Bauman and Dent (1982) found increased self-reporting among adolescents who had smoked recently when they were informed about the biologic measure before self-reporting. More recently, Murray, O'Connell, Schmidt, and Perry (1987), in a survey of 770 adolescents, found that twice as many students with elevated CO levels reported smoking under the bogus pipeline procedure. Consequently the use of biochemical validation became almost necessary in federally funded research.

Other researchers have shown that adolescents can report accurately when sufficient assurance of confidentiality is stressed. Williams, Eng, Botvin, Hill, and Ernst (1979) found that 98% of the adolescents who reported never smoking had nondetectable plasma cotinine levels. Murray and Perry (1987) found increased disclosure by manipulating conditions, including believable anonymity, the pipeline procedure, or both, with little difference found between the three groups. They assert, "It appears that smokers who might be persuaded to acknowledge their tobacco use are brought to that admission by either manipulation alone" (p. 231), at least in cross-sectional studies. A very careful explanation of tracking procedures and guarantee of anonymity is needed to ensure honest reports in longitudinal studies. Murray and Perry question whether confidentiality is possible in longitudinal studies.

Hansen, Mallotte, and Fielding (1985) did not find differences in self-reports between bogus pipeline and simple confidentiality conditions in previously measured youths. In fact, subjects who were asked to provide specimens reacted negatively to the biologic monitoring, and a sizable portion refused to participate. It seems that longitudinal bogus pipeline procedures may be more detrimental than useful. Thus use of a confidentiality procedure is likely to be just as worthwhile as use of a pipeline procedure in longitudinal research.

In Stacy, Flay, Sussman, Brown, et al. (1990), the convergent validity of popularly used open-ended versus closed-ended self-report measures of smoking was examined in a sample of 741 eleventh-grade Canadian high school students. Carbon monoxide (CO) samples were obtained as an independent method of assessing recent smoking. Along with CO, six known psychosocial correlates of smoking measured on closed-ended self-report scales (attitude, intention, subjective norms, risk taking, best friend's smoking, and other friends' smoking) were employed in bivariate analyses to estimate convergence with the self-report smoking indices. The results indicated that both simple ordinal scales of self-reported cigarette use, with only a few response options, and more continuous measures performed about equally as well as correlates of CO and the psychosocial measures, but only if the open-ended scales were subjected to a normalizing transformation to optimize their convergence.

Dent, Sussman, Stacy, Burton, and Flay (in preparation) found that use of a CO measure in the classroom will elicit elevated reports of smokeless tobacco use relative to nonuse of a CO measure, even though smokeless tobacco use cannot actually be detected through CO measurement. The Dent et al. study and other research (Freir, Bell, & Ellickson, 1991) suggest that the main problem in tobacco use measurement is a false positive rate. More specifically, adolescents tend to use tobacco too infrequently for use to be detected by a biochemical (objective) standard. Contrary to what might be found with adult tobacco users, the false negative rate (i.e., report of nonuse, but tobacco metabolites are detected through use of a biochemical device) is low. Possibly, infrequent users believe that their tobacco use will be detected by any biochemical device, and this is why they report relatively elevated rates of use.

In summary, a simple self-report measure of tobacco use and under conditions of anonymity will produce maximum reports of use. Under conditions of confidentiality, any type of biochemical validation will maximize self-reports of tobacco use. As a side note, given the human subjects issue of deception, now researchers uniformly make use of a "pipeline" (not bogus pipeline) procedure, in which subsamples of youth actually do receive biochemical validation of their reports. Finally, with adolescents and adults, recent studies suggest little advantage of collecting more expensive cotinine data over CO data (Dent et al., in preparation; Murray, Connett, Lauger, & Voelker, 1993).

Peculiarities in the Measurement of Smokeless Tobacco Use

Even though biochemical validation can be used as a corroborator or as a correlate of self-reports of smokeless tobacco use, it remains difficult even to measure quantities of smokeless tobacco used. Smokeless tobacco varies in forms and use size. Number of times used probably is the easiest means to gauge use. More specific data are as follows. Data from Gritz et al. (1981) indicate a use pattern of dipping/chewing an average of 8.8 (SD = 2.1) wads/day for a mean of 24.2 (SD = 4.3) minutes/wad at a mean interval of 85 (*SD* = 2.4) minutes (*n* = 12; age mean = 19). Consumption was an average of 10.8 (*SD* = 2.4) grams (31.6% of a can) of moist ground snuff on the experimental day, which did not differ from a self-report of average daily consumption (mean = 15.3, *SD* = 3.0 g; 45% of a can).

Data from Eakin, Severson, and Glasgow (1989) indicate a use pattern in which the number of dips per day was 10, with a can lasting a mean of 5 days. A dip was kept in the mouth just under 1 hour, and the mean weight of a dip was 1.2 grams (range 0.1-7.3 g; *n* = 84; mean age = 32; very wide variation in responses). Data from Williams (1975) on high school students reveal that 84% of the students dip only once per day (*n* = 220), with a duration of around 30 minutes (70%). Nicotine levels vary from Copenhagen (30.7 mg/g) to Kodiak (14 mg/g), Skoal (10.7 mg/g), and Hawkin or Skoal Bandits (approximately 5.7 mg/g; Severson, 1992). Putting the available data together suggests that young adult and regular snuff users will use about 1.2 grams nine times per day and exhaust a can in around 3 days. Also, they will move to higher-nicotine-containing brands over time (recall data reported in Chapter 1). Users of chewing tobacco may use less, perhaps even 50% less per day. However, more research is needed on chewers.

SCHOOL PERSONNEL INTERVIEWS

One simple method of estimating school-level student use would be to obtain estimates from school personnel. School personnel are likely to be well aware of school tobacco use norms (Evans et al., 1979). Personnel could be asked what percentage of the students at the whole school, or from a specific grade if certain grades are being targeted for programming, have tried or regularly use a tobacco product. The accuracy of this method was first reported by Charlin et al. (1990), as summarized later in this chapter. This type of data takes at most only 2 days to collect and analyze; the data collected could be quite detailed if collected through one-on-one interviews, students are not assessed directly so that reactivity is minimal, and the total cost of data collection from six individuals at one school would be only about $130. Teachers, counselors, administrators, janitors, coaches, and other personnel (such as cafeteria workers or secretarial support staff) who may be familiar with school drug use patterns are usually interviewed.

School personnel reports enable respondents to communicate not only their knowledge of student tobacco use but also their knowledge of the school social context. Due to time constraints of those who are interviewed (during the working day) and for ease of data analysis, interviews often take the form of self-administered questionnaires, an advantage of this form of interview being the potential to eliminate interviewer bias (Kidder, 1981). The effects of bias also are reduced by standardizing the interview. Questions generally consist of a combination of fixed-alternative and of open-ended types.

Results of Project TNT School Personnel Interview Study

Project TNT interviewed 378 staff members in the fall of 1987 from 30 junior high schools (15 rural, 15 urban) and 24 high schools (12 in southern California, 12 in Illinois). Twenty-three percent were principals or vice-principals, 10% were custodians, 40% were teachers, 16% were coaches and/or physical education teachers, 8% were counselors or clerical staff, and 3% were security officials or cafeteria workers. Interview content was aimed mainly at ascertaining facts, opinions, and beliefs regarding tobacco use in the school context—type of products and location of use, the interaction of use of smokeless tobacco with cigarettes, relationship of tobacco use to use of other drugs, school smoking policies for staff or for students, whether smoking rules are enforced, identification of adults who use, estimation of percentage of students and staff who use tobacco, and functions served by use of tobacco. Overall, staff reported that 46% of their students had tried cigarettes and that 12% were regular smokers (53% being males), whereas 12% of students had tried smokeless tobacco and 3% were regular users (91% being males). Staff were aware that the legal purchasing age for tobacco products in California is 18 years. As official policy, students were not permitted to use either tobacco substance on campus. To deter use of tobacco, they emphasized long-term consequences with students (78% and 75% for cigarettes and smokeless tobacco, respectively).

Staff varied widely about where students smoke cigarettes, although 19% and 11% said "at home" for cigarettes and smoke-less tobacco, respectively; 12% and 5% said "at parties"; 1% and 18% said "at athletic competitions"; 21% and 18% said "outdoors"; 27% and 11% said "near the school grounds"; and 28% and 13% said "to and from school." Sixty-eight percent reported that they had seen students smoking near the school (in the washrooms, 45%; at the sports fields, 20%; in the parking lots, 13%; in open/grounds areas, 19%; in areas near the school, 17%; and at "Ag" shops, 17%), and 25% reported that they had seen students using smokeless tobacco near the school (in the washrooms, 5%; at the sports fields, 15%; in the parking lots, 3%; in open/grounds areas, 6%; in areas near the school, 2%; and at "Ag" shops, 10%). Most staff thought students used tobacco after school (60%), though some thought before school as well (22%).

Staff reports of reasons their students use cigarettes and smokeless tobacco varied widely, but included to "look tough, risky" (19% for both), to be "popular/part of a group" (57% and 33% for cigarettes and smokeless tobacco, respectively), to "look mature" (36% and 15%), because "adults do" (19% and 12%), because they are pushed into it (16% and 10%), and because of "advertisements or that sports figures use it" (6% and 33%). In terms of why they thought students would choose smokeless tobacco over cigarettes, reasons included safety (21%), concealment (31%), ease of use (4%), and acceptability (3%).

The most popularly endorsed obstacles to quitting cigarettes and smokeless tobacco among students, according to these staff, included not receiving enough support from family and friends (19% and 18%), family and friends' use of tobacco (16% and 12%), lack of will power (12% and 10%), withdrawal symptoms (20% and 18%), and peer pressure (21% and 13%). Fifty-five percent and 37% reported that they believed their students would want to join a group that taught them to quit smoking or quit using smokeless tobacco, respectively.

Staff also gave reports about their own tobacco use behavior. Main reasons for staff first trial of cigarettes and smokeless tobacco, as reported among only those who had tried a tobacco product, included curiosity (44% and 50%) and tobacco use being an activity that they shared with others, (38% and 24%). Only 7% said they had been explicitly pushed into trying tobacco products, and these staff were those who did not become heavier users.

In terms of current cigarette or smokeless tobacco use self-reported by school staff (total ns = 61 and 6), 17% and 0% of the security officials or cafeteria workers (ns = 2 and 0); 16% and 1% of the teachers (ns = 24 and 2); 15% and 0% of the counselors or clerical staff (ns = 5 and 0); 12% and 1% of the administrators (ns = 10 and 1); 35% and 2% of the janitorial staff (ns = 13 and 1); and 12% and 3% of the coaches (ns = 7 and 2) were smokers and smokeless tobacco users, respectively. Of the respondents, 57% said that there was a formal smoking area (and rules) for staff; 27% said they had not seen staff smoking in or near the school; 45% saw smoking only in staff lounges; and 27% said they saw staff smoking at various places about the school. Half of the staff had been heavy lifetime smokers (over 99 cigarettes), although relatively few had been extensively involved in smokeless tobacco use (n = 6 used more than 99 times).

REFUSE ANALYSIS

Another method of obtaining information about student tobacco use at the school level is through use of garbage or household refuse analysis (garbology). Garbology is a contemporary anthropological technique based on methods used by archeologists for the study of past societies. In the framework of archeology and sociocultural anthropology, artifacts (the material system of a society) are reflections of the society's values, beliefs, and social structure (Rathje & Ritenbaum, 1984). These artifacts not only mirror people's actions and attitudes but, in the case of modern society, also shape them. Recently, behavioral scientists have begun to systematically observe artifacts in their behavioral context in today's culture. This has been done to supplement and evaluate traditional methods of data collection (Webb, Campbell, Schwartz, & Sechrest, 1966) and to provide a unique alternative perspective on the structure and content of our modern society. In the present context, by recording a count of tobacco refuse at schools, one may be able to provide an impersonal means of gauging school-level tobacco use. An exacting refuse collection procedure (Barovich, Sussman, Galaif, Dent, & Charlin, 1988) would take only one day to collect and analyze the data and would cost no more than $50. Clearly, this approach is the least time consuming and least expensive, and possibly would create the least reactivity, among the measures of tobacco use.

Refuse analysis estimates may be calculated by measuring areas surveyed (e.g., cigarette butts in parking lots) by use of a pedometer, producing a rough score of usage per square foot. Because of the likelihood that usage rates could be grossly exaggerated by a limited cleaning schedule, janitors are asked about the frequency with which areas to be surveyed—such as sports playing fields—are swept. Usage rates can then be compared across schools, regionally and individually. Interrater agreement generally is high (above .8).

Project TNT Refuse Analysis Study

Three methods of estimating school-level experimentation with tobacco products by adolescents were explored. Included in the study were 19 schools (5 urban and 8 rural junior high schools, and 3 urban and 3 rural high schools). Project TNT used Campbell and Fiske's (1959) criteria to estimate convergent and discriminant validity of a correlation matrix consisting of two "traits" (trial of cigarettes and smokeless tobacco) and three "methods" (aggregated student self-report, school personnel prevalence estimate, and school outdoor refuse evidence of tobacco products; also see Charlin, Sussman, Stacey et al., 1990 for details).

The *school personnel prevalence estimates* of student trial of tobacco products were collected from 124 school staff members (two administrators, two or three teachers, and two or three staff members at each school) using a structured interview. Assurances of confidentiality of the data were made, other detailed information was gathered, and the total time per interview was approximately 20 minutes.

Two observers (one male and one female) worked independently but at the same time at each school to *collect refuse data*. School observers were provided with "mapping areas" (see Barovich et al., 1988) that they had to follow in the process of collecting the data. The maps were a routing sequence of the locations to be examined. Three specific sites were inspected, following the same sequence at each school. The sites were (a) the parking lot (in high schools, the student parking lot was examined), (b) the sports field (that area where baseball and football are played most frequently), and (c) the "hangout" area (the site identified by staff as where students congregate during off-class hours).

The observers were instructed to search for any evidence of refuse of tobacco product use, particularly smokeless tobacco and cigarettes. The types of evidence that were recorded were entered under the column "Evidence Type" on a recording sheet and included items such as cans, wrappers, leaf, plug, and pouches for smokeless tobacco use, and butts, wrappers, and packages for smoking cigarettes. Each entry (presence of evidence) recorded on the form at each site for the different evidence item types was considered a separate "instance." A total of 133 different instances of tobacco product refuse was found. The agreement among observers, evaluated using a Pearson correlation between the counts from both observers, was $r = .95$ across all types of evidence ($r = .74$ for smokeless tobacco, and $r = .94$ for cigarette evidence). Given the high agreement among observers, an average of the counts from both observers was used as the count for the analyses. A general composite measure was developed from the sum of all counts for both tobacco products in the parking lots, the sports field, and the "hangout" areas. This measure was adjusted for the size of the areas examined and the number of students at the school. Thus the two measures corresponded to evidence of smokeless tobacco and cigarette refuse per student per square yard, respectively.

Student trial of tobacco products was assessed with either structured *interviews* to 198 students or a *survey* administered to 1,170 students. These data were collected as part of other project studies, and involved assessments of an average of 75% of the students enrolled within each of three classrooms from each school. This item was coded as proportion of 7th (or 10th) graders who ever tried the tobacco product at that school.

Results and Discussion

The student self-report and school staff report methods demonstrated good convergent validity ($r = .67$ for cigarettes, $.54$ for smokeless tobacco). The refuse method showed convergent validity with student self-reports of smokeless tobacco use ($r = .54$) but not with self-reports of smoking ($r = .12$). Refuse and school personnel reports were not significantly correlated ($rs < .30$). We found a trend toward discriminant validity for the aforementioned relations. We suggest that, of the three methods, the school personnel prevalence estimate is the most useful and economic one for estimating school-level tobacco experimentation. The refuse method is valuable as a means to rank schools on prevalence of student tobacco use, particularly regarding smokeless tobacco use.

NATURALISTIC OBSERVATION

Naturalistic observation provides an alternative approach to studying adolescent tobacco use situations. Naturalistic observation, though not a well-developed method in adolescent tobacco use studies, is fairly common in ethology, zoology, and anthropology (e.g., Sackett, 1978). This method involves (a) the recording of events in their natural settings at the time they occur, (b) the use of trained impartial observers, and (c) descriptions of behaviors and events that require little if any inference to code (Jones, Reid, & Patterson, 1975). This method can be difficult to implement because adolescent smoking often takes place in private and is illegal (Biglan, Weissman, & Severson, 1985). On the other hand, it is not uncommon to observe teenagers smoking in public settings.

The potential benefit of the approach is that a behavioral event can be observed as it occurs. In this sense, it is less subject to subjective report bias. Of course, naturalistic observation is subject to observer bias. Observer bias is minimized by operationalizing target behavior so as to require minimal inferences and by establishing interrater agreement (Sackett, 1978). Lofland (1971) cautions, however, that in being concerned with occurrences, types, possibilities, and details in qualitative observation, there is always the temptation to look for correlations. He suggests that in qualitative observation the most that can be done is to report suggestions and impressions about frequency and correlation.

Project TNT Naturalistic Observation Study

A naturalistic observation study of adolescent tobacco use was conducted to corroborate previous studies that used self-report questionnaire or structured interview methods to study this problem behavior (see Sussman, Hahn, Dent, Stacy, et al., 1993, for details). A stratified, random selection procedure was used to select 16 schools in southern California. A total of 4 urban junior high schools, 6 rural junior high schools, 3 urban high schools, and 3 rural high schools were selected from a pool of 100 schools. These schools consisted of equal numbers of males and females and equal numbers of students from urban and rural areas. Ethnicity did not differ between schools: 70% were white, 20% were Hispanic, 5% were black, and 5% were Asian.

All of the observations were conducted by three experienced raters. The observers were instructed to search for tobacco use at the schools in places named as "hangout spots" by school personnel (Charlin et al., 1990). In addition, the observers searched in the student parking lots, then drove around the campus in circles that widened by one block with each rotation, to a three-block radius. Observations were made in the morning during the 30 minutes before school began, at lunchtime for a 30-minute period, and for the first 30 minutes after school let out. When use was found, the observers remained as inconspicuous as possible; situations observed were recorded after the observer was out of sight of the users, many of the observations were made from the observers' automobiles, and observers located themselves 15 feet or more away from the students. Students were not approached during the study.

Measure

A single-sheet checklist-type instrument was developed to minimize visibility of the observations and to maximize speed of
completion. Observers first noted on a space provided their distance from the tobacco users or tobacco-using groups, assigning a
letter to each student in the group (A, B, C, and so on), and
diagramming each student's position. Observers used the letters
to identify each student when completing items that were presented in the checklist format. Items rated in this checklist included the student's ethnic group, sex, apparent age, clothing
style, dominant facial expression, substance being used (cigarette,
smokeless tobacco, other, none), offer being made to others, refusal or acceptance of offer, and other notable behavior (e.g.,
passing the same cigarette). Likely accuracy of age estimates was
established in a pilot study (see Barovich, Sussman, Dent, Burton,
& Flay, 1991). In that pilot study, interrater agreement was quite
high ($r = .95$), and the age ratings did not differ significantly from
each other or from self-reported age of 30 targeted young people
(all three $ts < 0.6$, $ps > .1$). Prior to collecting the data presented
here, the raters independently rated 10 high school students so-
cializing in three small groups at a high school. Interrater reliability collapsed across categories was high with no training (average
$r = .82$).

Results and Discussion

Observers conducted 48 searches for use in the fall of 1987 (3 per
school) and observed 15 different use situations (which involved
a total of 41 youths). Eleven of the 15 situations were observed
after school, one before school, and three at lunchtime. The 15
observations occurred at six schools; five were high schools. Female subjects constituted 46% of the sample. Ages were estimated
as being between 13 and 18 years old. Of the students observed,
80% were white, 10% were Hispanic, 8% were black, and 2% were
Asian. All observations of smoking in groups took place on the
school grounds; two observations of individual's smoking took
place within one-half block of school. Each situation had between
1 and 10 subjects, with the mean number of students in each group

being 3 (SD = 2.8 students). Nine students were alone. The other 32 students were grouped as follows: one group of 3 females, one group of 3 males, two groups of 5 students of mixed sexes (2 males and 3 females), one group of 6 males, and one group of 10 students of mixed sexes (5 males and 5 females). Seven offers of tobacco were observed in two situations—one within a group of 5 students and the other within a group of 10 students. Four of these offers were between students who were sharing the same cigarette. No refusals of tobacco were detected by the observers. One request for a cigarette was observed in the group of 10 students. Five students lit their cigarettes from another student's cigarette in this group. All of the situations observed were of cigarette use. No smokeless tobacco use or any other drug use was observed.

Results converged with certain findings from more traditional questionnaire and interview methods of studying adolescent tobacco use (e.g., as summarized by Flay et al., 1983). Each method reports that many youth smoke cigarettes in small groups, which involve sharing cigarettes and making offers to use. Still, some differences among findings based on these alternative methods are evident. The naturalistic observation approach, relative to the others, identified a small percentage of offers to smoke, revealed groups containing both users and nonusers, and found more solitary use. Perhaps less emphasis should be placed on assertion refusal training in prevention programming, and more emphasis should be placed on informational sources of social influence to use tobacco (Sussman, 1989). Theories of informational social influence, such as observational learning through modeling (Bandura, 1977), emphasize the *inferential* processes resulting from the observation of others' behavior, rather than direct social pressure.

Of those observed, 22% were alone when using tobacco, compared to 12% reported through interviews of junior high and high school students (Hahn et al., 1990). Instances observed at school relative to other contexts may reflect an overrepresentation of older students, who more openly display their use of tobacco. Solitary smokers were among the oldest youth observed, with all but one being estimated to be 17 years of age or older. Those who were observed smoking alone may be heavier smokers and may have nicotine cravings that they satisfy even when the group is not available. Alternatively, some youth may not develop tobacco use in group situations. It is possible that the students observed smoking alone began smoking for personal reasons, such as to relieve boredom or stress (Wills, 1986) or to experience pleasure (Bauman & Chenowith, 1984). Research on solitary versus group-based smoking among adolescents is needed.

ARCHIVAL DATA

Along with self-report, refuse, school personnel, and naturalistic observation data, archival data have been used to identify smoking-related school dimensions. Skager and Fisher (1994) used archival data along with self-report data and found that schools that were primarily white, rural, and small-sized or white, urban, high-SES, and large-sized were at greater risk for drug use. Dent, Sussman, and Flay (1993) used a previous institute project data set (Project TVSFP; Flay et al., 1988), and also collected concurrent archival school-level data from the California Department of Education. Archival data collected included grade enrollment; number of classes in the grade (6th grade); total number of grades at the school; ethnic composition; percentage of students with English as a second language (ESL); socioeconomic status; percentage of students receiving aid (AFDC); and reading, writing, and math California Achievement Program (CAP) scores. With these data they replicated an earlier study that used such data to demonstrate use of a randomized blocking procedure to assign a small number of units to conditions (Graham, Flay, Johnson, Hansen, & Collins, 1984). Also, using factor loadings of these archival data, Dent, Sussman, and Flay (1993) projected student tobacco and other drug use onto a factor analysis solution space. They found that mean lifetime tobacco use was higher in schools that were largely white, academically high achieving, smaller in size, and lower in public assistance. Different relations were found regarding use of other substances, however. For example, intention to use alcohol was higher in larger, minority-dominated schools. Archival data used to select and assign schools in Project TNT were presented in Chapter 5 of this book, and included U.S. Census data as well as California Department of Education data. These data sources remain reliable sources of corroborative data regarding correlates of tobacco use at the school or zipcode level. Recent California statewide data provides reasonable county-level estimates of tobacco use among adolescents (Burns & Pierce, 1992).

STORE PERSONNEL INTERVIEWS AND OBSERVATION

To enhance tobacco use prevention efforts, it is important to better understand the situational factors that promote use. One important, but mostly neglected, situational factor is the presence of stores that promote tobacco use near schools. Most experimentation with tobacco products, including both cigarettes and smokeless tobacco, occurs right after school lets out (Hahn et al., 1990), and stores provide ready access to tobacco products (Kirn, 1987; Forster, Klepp, & Jeffery, 1989). Stores located near schools undoubtedly are frequented by youth on their way to and from school and may be utilized as "hangout" areas. Store personnel at those stores may sell tobacco products to minors and openly model tobacco use. Tobacco products are prominently displayed in stores, which may enhance adolescent curiosity to try tobacco products. A more complete understanding of the role of store policy and store personnel behavior regarding tobacco sales and use near the store could help further prevention efforts to address this important situational influence on tobacco use.

Braverman et al. (1989) examined the marketing of smokeless tobacco at 199 stores in 13 counties in California by recording information about products located on the shelves in these stores. They found that large cities in rural counties and small towns in urban counties had the highest availability of smokeless tobacco products, particularly moist snuff. Large cities in urban counties had the lowest availability of tobacco products, suggesting, contrary to what might be expected, that availability does not increase simply with increasing community size or urbanicity. Sales inducements were more present in urban stores, perhaps as an attempt to promote use in some lower sales areas.

Alternative types of data would permit a more complete assessment of availability and sales of tobacco products to adolescents at stores. Recent research utilizing self-report data and adolescent "confederates" at stores have provided good evidence that store owners will sell cigarettes to minors (Altman, Foster, Rasinick-Doussi, & Tye, 1989). No study though, has provided interviews of store personnel sufficiently detailed to address employees' own behavior and attitudes, and no study has tried to complement such interviews with naturalistic observations of tobacco-purchasing behavior by youth.

Project TNT Store Personnel Study

We investigated availability of tobacco products to adolescents at those stores located closest to public junior high and high schools by using three methods: (a) interviewing store personnel (one per store); (b) recording types and location of tobacco products, promotional items, and the legal age warning signs within stores; and (c) observing purchasing behavior (Barovich et al., 1991). Stores were selected through use of a randomized block design. Specifically, stores were yoked to schools that were picked through use of a stratified random selection procedure. Store personnel were interviewed at randomly selected southern California ($n = 36$) and Illinois stores ($n = 12$).

Results and Discussion

Results showed that store personnel used tobacco at twice the rate of the general public. Although only two people (7% of the sample) reported themselves as having been heavy lifetime users of smokeless tobacco, high percentages of southern California and Illinois personnel reported themselves to be current smokers (61% in southern California and 67% in Illinois), twice as high as the national average of 28% (Pierce, 1989). They also reported that they often used tobacco while working at the store.

At 19 of 36 southern California stores, smokeless tobacco *products* were placed on or behind the cash register at the counter, and those products were placed in that location in most Illinois stores (9 of 12). In over half the stores, they were placed in more than one location—if not on the counter, then by other tobacco products or candy. Smokeless tobacco look-alike products were present at 58% of the stores in southern California and at 33% of the Illinois stores. Most frequently, the product was gum contained in chewing-tobacco-like packages (e.g., Big League Chew). Smokeless tobacco promotional items (coupons, order forms, displays, and posters) were present at 55% of the stores in southern California and at 42% of the stores in Illinois.

A variety of data provided in this study suggest that stores proximal to schools serve as a primary site for adolescent tobacco acquisition and experimentation. Approximately half of the store employees in southern California and Illinois said they would sell tobacco products to minors if "they were buying it for their parents." These results corroborate our earlier observations (Sussman, 1987) and the observations of Connolly (Kirn, 1987), who found that a 14-year-old girl was able to successfully purchase cigarettes at 75% of the stores she visited. Apparently, a majority of convenience stores will sell cigarettes to minors. The present study (Barovich et al., 1991) not only corroborates those results but extends them; many store personnel will admit that they sell these products to minors, while knowing that this practice is illegal, when the questionnaire item is worded, "Do you sell [tobacco] to minors if they say they're buying it for their parents?" Further, several apparently illegal purchases were observed. The purchase observation data from this study suggests that one can expect to observe at least one illegal tobacco sale during the hour that school lets out at those stores closest to schools.

Almost all purchases observed were of cigarettes. However, a nationally documented increase in sales of smokeless tobacco (as well as the increase in sales reported in our sample) may be accounted for by an increase in the purchase of smokeless tobacco by youth, because the largest increase in sales of smokeless tobacco has been to those under 18 years of age (Sussman, 1989). Possibly, sales of smokeless tobacco products generally are more infrequent than those of cigarettes, or sales tend to occur primarily at times other than those that were observed.

Adolescents do "hang out" in and around convenience stores. Many of these stores serve a recreational purpose. As observed anecdotally by data collectors, several stores appeared to be congregating points for numerous young people, many of whom were playing video games. The availability of tobacco products, snack foods, alcohol, magazines, and video games (for entertainment purposes) must seem desirable to some youths. While at the store, even for a brief period, youth inevitably will observe the presence of tobacco products; these products are prominently displayed. Yet laws regarding the legal age for purchase of tobacco generally are not posted (they were posted at only 5 of 48 stores in the present study), even though the state law requires posting of warning labels for cash registers and store windows stating that it is illegal to sell cigarettes or chewing tobacco to anyone under the age of 18. Further, one may speculate that because store personnel use twice as much tobacco as the general public (Pierce, 1989), stores are a major site for observation of tobacco use by adolescents while away from their parents.

SUMMARY OF MEASURES USED IN PROJECT TNT OUTCOMES STUDY

To assign schools to conditions in a randomized block design, Project TNT used students tobacco use reports, school personnel reports, and archival data to define blocks. To measure implementation and process, the project used student, classroom teacher-observer, and Project TNT health educator self-reports. To measure tobacco use outcomes, Project TNT used a biochemical pipeline procedure for a confidential data collection cohort, and an anonymous procedure for a grade-level-defined cohort. Thus Project TNT used multiple approaches, including many described in this chapter. Project TNT did not use refuse analysis, naturalistic observation, or store personnel interviews as measures in the main outcomes trial, or use school personnel reports at follow-up time points, viewing them as still in need of more refinement to make sure they are useful as measures to assign schools to conditions or gauge tobacco use outcomes. Further, project monetary resources limited making use of all possible available types of measures.

PART THREE

Curriculum Development, Implementation, and Follow-Up in Prevention

Part Three provides detailed information on curriculum development, implementation and outcomes evaluation in prevention—often not discussed in health education research (Sussman, 1991). Chapter 7 describes the method of curriculum development used by Project TNT. Chapter 8 focuses on the final curricula contents and implementation of the curricula, questionnaire development and contents, and data collection. Finally, Chapter 9 presents the implementation, process, and outcomes evaluation of the prevention component of Project TNT.

SEVEN

Curriculum Development Applied to Prevention in Project TNT

On the basis of previous theoretical or empirical work (e.g., Atkins, 1978; Evans, Raines, & Owen, 1989; Flay, 1986; Flay et al., 1988; Kliebard, 1989; Kunstel, 1978) and the experiences in curriculum development by Project TNT, four general steps of curriculum development are suggested for use in school-based prevention research (Sussman, 1991). These four steps were applied by Project TNT. The first step involves *adopting and extending a theoretical knowledge base,* and includes adoption of a theoretical perspective, and use of assessment studies to increase theoretically relevant knowledge regarding variables that facilitate or deter risk behavior. Application of the first, theoretically-oriented step was described in earlier chapters. The second step is one of *pooling curriculum activities,* and involves collecting previously used curriculum activities and teaching methods from other projects in related areas that have obtained research support and might be useful in the present curriculum development context. This step also involves development of new activities that are hypothesized to counteract certain antecedent variables. The third step involves *testing of individual activities* and may include the use of (a) theme studies or focus groups to explore the perceived interest and efficacy of proposed classroom activities or full lessons, followed by (b) experimental or quasi-experimental studies (component studies)

(Step 1)
CREATE A KNOWLEDGE BASE
[Theory as a guide]
Assessment studies to gather more information
↓
(Step 2)
POOL CURRICULA ACTIVITIES
[Plausible counteraction of an etiological factor]
Derive from old curricula or develop new activities
↓
(Step 3)
TEST INDIVIDUAL ACTIVITIES
[To provide a means of assessing counteraction on an etiological factor]
Theme studies, focus groups, component studies
↓
(Step 4)
CREATE AND TEST A COMPLETE CURRICULUM
[To create an internally consistent package that counteracts an etiological factor]
Lesson building, feasibility study, pilot study

Figure 7.1. Curriculum Development Process
SOURCE: Adapted from Sussman, 1991.

to examine the immediate effects of a program activity or full
lesson on knowledge, attitudes, or behavioral intentions. The
fourth and final step involves *testing of a full curriculum,* which
includes (a) combining activities and lessons to produce a curriculum, (b) feasibility ("soft data") studies to assess the general
workability and sequencing of curriculum lessons and, finally, (c)
pilot studies, which provide pretest and posttest ratings of a whole
curriculum delivered to multiple classrooms. These steps are described in more detail as follows, and are illustrated in Figure 7.1.

POOLING CURRICULUM ACTIVITIES

Once a decision has been made about which paradigm or paradigm combination to use as a theoretical guide, and about engaging in additional assessment studies to complete gaps in knowledge
regarding the risk behavior, the next step is to collect school-based
curriculum activities and teaching methods that have proven

useful in previous research, as well as to create new activities. Important material to be considered for the construction of a curriculum includes (a) number and scheduling of program lessons, and (b) typical activities and teaching methods used in a curriculum.

Number and Scheduling of Lessons

In previous research, particularly in drug abuse and cigarette smoking prevention studies, the number of lessons delivered has ranged from 4 to 20. Programs with as few as 5 lessons have been successful in delaying drug use onset (Evans, 1976; Evans et al., 1978; Hurd et al., 1980; McAlister, 1983), and it is possible that delivery of a daily program is superior to a more intermittent presentation (Botvin, Renick, & Baker, 1983). More research is needed here. Instruction of a whole curriculum is more critical than the spacing of lessons. Instruction of only a subset of lessons is likely to result in an ineffective program.

It is clear that booster lessons may significantly enhance program effects, especially when repeated over a number of years (Flay et al., 1989), and these have been a feature in advanced-generation primary prevention studies (e.g., Flay, 1985, 1987a). Messages that are repeated over relatively long periods of time and that allow expression of newly formed attitudes and behaviors are relatively likely to be incorporated into one's personal repertoire (Flay, 1981; Flay et al., 1983); thus a reasonably inclusive booster period for each curriculum seems appropriate (Botvin et al., 1983; Flay et al., 1985). Of course, schools do not usually allow booster periods longer than one week. Therefore treatment delivery might be maximized if programs were delivered at two or more time points during a period when a risk behavior tends to increase, including perhaps 5 to 10 core lessons and 1 to 5 booster lessons taught 6 months to one year later, and ideally throughout adolescence (Flay et al., 1989), allowing integration of program material with daily life experiences in between each set, and a sufficient number of total lessons (i.e., at least seven; Glynn, 1989; Silvestri & Flay, 1989).

Activity Pool

Several types of activities or approaches toward teaching are typically used to impart substantive material in a curriculum (e.g., Anderson & Creswell, 1976, pp. 238-248, discuss 43 specific types of activities). Four main classes of teaching methods or activities used in many of the school-based tobacco use primary prevention projects are (a) the Socratic method and use of peer leaders to teach substantive material; (b) social skills training, involving modeling, behavioral rehearsal, role play, or viewing videotapes; (c) writing and group activities to encourage belief change and to obtain a statement of personal commitment not to engage in the risk behavior (e.g., letter writing, videotaping public commitment); and (d) extra-training involvement activities to personalize information and extend the contexts and agents of preventive efforts (e.g., homework, discussions with family). The research support for these activities is described below (also see Sussman, 1991).

Use of the Socratic Method and Peer Leaders

The Socratic method of teaching is one whereby questioning by the teacher is used to elicit from participants the pertinent prevention information. This process is preferable to the didactic approach because it reduces resistance to the message and encourages discussion and consensus among group members (e.g., Flay et al., 1988).

Peers may more effectively learn social skills or other information from each other, or from older students, than from adults (e.g., Young et al., 1988). On the other hand, adults may appear more credible and provide better lesson implementation. Although results are not consistent (Clarke et al., 1986; Johnson, 1982; McCaul & Glasgow, 1985), it appears that the involvement of peers as behavioral models for classmates may be helpful. This does not necessarily involve having peers lead class activities.

Social Skills Training

Those who engage in risk behaviors including drug use have been found to demonstrate poorer social skills, at least assertion refusal skill, than those who do not engage in such behavior (e.g., Reardon et al., 1989; Wills, Baker, & Botvin, 1989). The objective of social skills training is to teach different skills (e.g., assertion refusal, communication skills) using a well-researched method. Essential components of skills training are described elsewhere (Bellack & Hersen, 1977; DeArmas & Brigham, 1986). Apparently, assertion refusal improvement in school-based programs is due to both learning and practice deficits, not teacher demand effects (Turner et al., 1993). Refusal assertion is discussed in detail in the component study section of this chapter.

Writing Exercises and Group Activities

Engaging students in writing exercises (e.g., letter writing) in the classroom and as homework may help them to personalize knowledge and become active learners (Tow & Smith, 1988). Various classroom group activities, such as those that involve taking of class polls, can effect conservative shifts in attitudes of class members (e.g., Hansen, Graham, et al., 1988). As an example, one activity ("normative restructuring") involves having the classroom divide up into groups defined by standing in front of a sign that indicates "approval" or "disapproval" of tobacco use. Most of the class will stand in front of the "disapproval" sign. Students learn that other class members hold attitudes as conservative as their own. They may shift in a conservative direction their previously held attitude about same-aged peer acceptance of tobacco use.

Extra-Training Involvement

Homework assignments are used regularly in school-based programs to (a) encourage review and generalization of training from one setting to another (e.g., school to home), and (b) expand the targets of the intervention (e.g., to siblings and parents). Research has shown that extra-training involvement can attain a suitable level (e.g., around 70% parental assistance in completing homework; Brannon et al., 1989). Parental involvement or involvement of the mass media or other community activities also is important to monopolize the youth's learning environment with pro-health information, and to supplement the material being learned at the school (e.g., Sussman, Brannon, et al., 1986; Sussman, Flay, et al., 1989).

New Activities

In addition to pooling well-researched curriculum activities, the researcher may need to develop fresh approaches. Sometimes activities from other contexts may not work well in a new context. Alternatively, a new activity conceptually may seem to more effectively counteract some antecedent variable.

The researcher is ready to go on to the third step of this development process only when multiple activities to counteract each major antecedent have been conceptualized. The purpose of subsequent steps is to contrast alternative activities that might counteract an antecedent variable, select the activity that has the strongest impact on mediators of change, refine the activity for use in a lesson, and then combine activities to build the curriculum.

TESTING INDIVIDUAL ACTIVITIES: THEME, FOCUS GROUP, AND COMPONENT STUDIES

The goal of the third step in curriculum development is to provide empirical validation of alternative activities. Various methodological approaches should be used to contrast curriculum activities regarding their ability to inhibit precursors of risk behavior. However, activities should be retained to compose a draft curriculum only if they (a) are guided by a specific theory, (b) are found to elicit knowledge change, (c) have a relatively favorable effect on attitudes and behavioral intentions (and do not affect these measures negatively), and (d) are perceived as relatively interesting by students.

The researcher could select activities from a subset of the methods described below due to time or cost considerations. However, a two-step sequence should be taken to help select an activity. One should begin by first doing either theme studies or focus groups, within which a large number of activities should be tested for their perceived impact. One should then proceed to do component studies, which are more costly but within which knowledge and attitude change can be detected. Each of these approaches has its own specific strengths and weaknesses, which are described so that the researcher can select the type of (a) perceived impact study (theme study or focus group) and (b) subsequent immediate impact study (component study) most relevant to his or her pursuits. The ideal research protocol would involve a combination of methods to provide convergent sources of validation for an activity.

Theme Studies

Theme studies consist of brief written descriptions of prevention activities, which are rated for their perceived interest and efficacy, and which provide a first active step toward writing the curriculum (Sussman, 1991; Sussman, Galaif, et al., 1989). Theme studies are of at least two types. One type consists of student-generated activities to counteract key acquisition variables. Specifically, students within a class are divided into groups, and each group is asked to develop a written description of an activity to counteract an acquisition variable presented by the researcher (e.g., smoking because a student thinks that everyone smokes). The students return to their desks, and a representative from each group reads the activity that his or her group generated (e.g., having the results of a large self-report survey read to the class). The students then provide ratings of each activity's "silliness," "interest," and "helpfulness" (for not engaging in the risk behavior). A second type of theme study consists of experimenter-generated activities to counteract acquisition variables, presented as written paragraphs that the students then rate using the same types of scales.

Strengths and Weaknesses

The potential strengths of the student-generated approach are that (a) students generate activities that are relevant to them, and (b) new activities are relatively likely to be generated. The strengths of the second approach are that (a) more standardization of the procedure is maintained across classrooms, and (b) it is possible to rate more activities per unit time. The strength of both approaches is that they allow for an empirical evaluation of many proposed activities. The obvious weakness of these approaches is that judgments are made of an activity's perceived efficacy, rather than the activity's actually being tried. Also, a further limitation of the second approach is that it is up to the discretion of the researcher and health educator to determine exactly which activities to evaluate. Theme studies help the researcher to select which activities might be most fruitfully tested, considering that cost and time limitations necessitate the completion of a very finite number of component or pilot studies.

Application to Project TNT

Project TNT tested both self-generated and experimenter-generated types of theme studies. In general, the self-generated activities were reported as slightly more fun, less silly, clear, and helpful than were the health-educator-generated activities. Still, the subjects seemed to understand the ratings. Several self-generated paragraph themes overlapped with the experimenter-generated ones, and we were able to select relatively good activities from both types of approaches.

Procedural suggestions from a summary report of the theme studies were incorporated into subsequent pilot studies. Students preferred certain activities to impart prevention information. These included interviewing of smokers as an activity and homework assignment; role playing of tobacco-use-related situations; skits to act out physical or social consequences; using imagination for physical or social consequences; use of a mirror primarily to increase self-esteem; and creating raps, guessing games, plays, and movies to impart prevention information. We also found that (a) an effort would have to be made to take students' focus off physical consequences information in the two social-influence-only curricula because some tendency for students to generate activities with this type of focus was noted; (b) students like to be actively involved in all lessons, either viewing behavior of others, or acting out tasks; they don't like simple lectures or class discussions; (c) ingratiation role plays, avoidance planning, refusal assertion, and activism strategies were preferred (perceived as the most interesting and helpful and the least "silly") for the normative social influence curriculum; (d) general conversation skills, self-esteem and debating skills, a focus on awareness of school groups who use tobacco, and social images modification were preferred for the informational social influence curriculum; (e) it appeared that role-playing having a disease and guided imagery activities were well received (e.g., imagining the toll of tobacco use on one's body through paired-image association tasks), but that more work was needed on making the addiction process understood if it was to be used in the physical consequences curriculum in the future; and (f) a reasonable listening skill/course involvement exercise was one where a person left the room and people had to recall what the person was wearing.

Focus Groups

Focus group methodology is one of the most widely used qualitative research tools in the applied social sciences (Basch, 1987; Stewart & Shamdasani, 1990). This approach has been described as applicable to various aspects of research, including exploratory or hypothesis generation, "clinical" uses (assessing respondents' nonverbal as well as verbal behavior), phenomenological uses (generating data within a group process-oriented setting), and confirmatory uses (interpreting results obtained through quantitative methods; Basch, 1987; Krueger, 1988; Morgan, 1988; Stewart & Shamdasani, 1990; Wimmer & Dominick, 1987). Recently this method has been proposed as a means to advance health education approaches (Basch, 1987; Stewart & Shamdasani, 1990); it has been used fruitfully in the development of adolescent tobacco use prevention (Heimann-Ratain, Hanson, & Peregoy, 1985; Parker et al., 1994; Worden et al., 1988) and cessation (Graham et al., 1993; Sussman, Burton, Dent, Stacy, & Flay, 1991) programs, and as a means to uncover reasons why youth drink and drive (Basch, DeCicco, & Malfetti, 1989).

Focus group procedures generally involve having a well-trained facilitator ask open-ended questions of a small group of 6 to 12 consumers. Research studies may use a standard format involving progressively more specific questions within the same group or successive groups. Most professional focus group moderators or research companies use what is known as an extended focus group procedure, which includes a pregroup questionnaire. The questionnaire encompasses material that will be covered during the session. Use of this questionnaire may help "commit" group members to a position before group discussion begins, so as to facilitate expression of minority as well as majority opinion during group discussion (Wimmer & Dominick, 1987).

Strengths and Weaknesses

This method is useful for generating activity information or for evaluating an activity described to the group, given the assumption that students know what they like and "what's good for them." Very in-depth information can be disclosed by this method, and answers given by students can be clarified through additional discussion. In addition, this technique may be a preferable one to use when tapping "sensitive" issues (e.g., AIDS or STD prevention) because a skillful group leader may reduce embarrassment and encourage openness about potentially threatening topics. In addition, the experimenter has more control over the group process than may be the case with other qualitative methods, such as participant observation. Group responses can be recorded and coded into a quantitative response system, or use of pretest and posttest questionnaires can supplement information gathered from the focus group (Basch, 1977; Krueger, 1988; Morgan, 1988; Stewart & Shamdasani, 1990; Wimmer & Dominick, 1987). However, the method's usefulness may be limited if no focus group replications are completed, and postgroup response coding and evaluation can be time consuming and difficult to evaluate (Evans et al., 1989). Furthermore, group consensus effects may lead to the elicitation of socially desirable (as opposed to completely honest) responses, and because of this the group process may not yield the types of content information that may be possible to obtain with an open-ended (and therefore confidential) questionnaire (Sussman et al., 1991).

Focus group researchers admit that group influence processes can distort individual opinion (thus necessitating use of the extended focus group procedure; Morgan, 1988; Wimmer & Dominick, 1987). Still, the impact of the focus group on responses of participating consumers rarely has been explored. One of the most well-researched group effects in the social sciences is that people will rely on the responses of other people, converging to a collective norm, given the operation of certain variables. "Collective norm" effects have been observed in studies involving manipulations of the autokinetic effect and studies of the risky shift phenomenon, group polarization, working groups, and psychotherapy groups (Eiser, 1980; Miles, 1981; Yalom, 1975). Focus groups, especially when used in health applications, contain many variables relevant to such judgment shifts, including that (a) the situation is relatively unstructured, (b) people identify their opinions (more than just discuss issues), (c) some people indicate agreement to a stated opinion, (d) people in the group know each other, and (e) group members are homogenous in composition (Basch, 1987; Eiser, 1980). Generally, subjects become more extreme in their judgments following group discussion (Sussman et al., 1991). A final weakness of focus groups is that subjects may tell more than they can know (Nisbett & Wilson, 1977). It is even possible that the most effective potential activity could be judged negatively in student focus group ratings. Thus focus groups should be used judiciously and should not necessarily override theoretical concerns. Also, the researcher should consider using both theme studies and focus groups, if possible, to obtain convergent validation of those activities that have the best perceived impact.

Application to Project TNT

Focus groups were used in the Project TNT prevention component as a means of generating the assessment studies used, and to clarify results obtained in the theme and component studies. We found focus groups very useful for idea generation and for clarification. As a curriculum development strategy, focus groups were used primarily for the cessation component because little is known about adolescent tobacco use cessation research. A discussion of use of focus groups for cessation program development is provided in Chapter 11.

Component Studies

At this point in the suggested curriculum development process, the researcher should have obtained perceived efficacy ratings and health educator judgments that suggest comparisons of activities to counteract the same acquisition variables. Multiple component studies should then be completed, each one contrasting two or more approaches toward a given program "component" (i.e., mediator of change). Component studies usually involve some experimental manipulation of several classrooms to two or more conditions (a between-groups or between-and-within groups design). A second type of component study design involves a simpler format of pretest, material presentation, and posttest, using baseline measures to provide a control for one or more classrooms (a one-group pretest-posttest design). These two types of methods have in common the development of a curriculum by testing variations in, or different, individual activities through a self-report assessment of activity process (e.g., involvement, perceived helpfulness) and immediate impact (e.g., changes in knowledge, attitudes, beliefs, intentions).

Different results are possible as a function of particular activity comparisons. Program activities may be differentially effective for different groups of youth (e.g., O'Neill et al., 1983), and some individual techniques may work best together to provide a maximal immediate preventive impact (e.g., Glasgow, McCaul, Freeborn, & O'Neill, 1981), or there may be a clear advantage of one type of manipulation over another (e.g., Sussman, Dent, Flay, et al., 1989). Thus it is optimal to contrast competing strategies within a fully crossed design to select the more effective strategy or combination of strategies.

Strengths and Weaknesses

Most previous curriculum development research in primary prevention has included component studies involving some experimental manipulation (McCaul & Glasgow, 1985). The strength of this approach is that one can manipulate potential mediators of change, allowing for selection of the best material for inclusion into a curriculum (McCaul & Glasgow, 1985). The potential weakness is that the activity or lesson is assessed without regard to other program activities, all of which, when combined, might add or detract from each other in achieving program effects. This approach also tends to be relatively expensive.

The alternative, one-group pretest-posttest design is both cost- and time-efficient and enables a thorough testing of curriculum components. Replications across different classrooms can be completed with promising activities that obtained equivocal results, leading to more refined activities. Unfortunately, a testing confound is possible, and no experimental manipulation is directly involved (Campbell & Stanley, 1973). Comparisons of activities can be accomplished through use of "matched" classrooms and/or assessments of the relative impact of different activities on process and immediate impact ratings obtained over several replications. In this way, subject selection effects can be controlled.

One is ready to begin to combine activities only when a sufficient number of activities have been tested: that is, (a) each activity retained has been found to be superior to at least one plausible alternative, (b) these activities manipulate proposed mediators of change (at least knowledge-related aspects), and (c) the number of component studies completed now permits creation of a complete curriculum.

Application to Project TNT

A total of 43 pretest-activity-posttest component studies were run to develop and refine Project TNT prevention curricula lessons, as summarized in Table 7.1. The primary outcome measures in these studies were ratings of learning, attention to the activity, and intention change. The outcomes of these activities are summarized as follows. Any significant increase in learning was indicated by "yes." Low attention to the activity was defined as less than 40% of the sample reporting interest in the activity, moderate interest was defined as 40% to 59% reporting interest, and high interest was defined as 60% or more reporting interest. Intention change was indicated by a shift in the responses of the sample. A 3% or greater shift toward decreased intention to use indicated a

Table 7.1 Component Studies Summary for Each Curriculum

Activity	Learning[a]	Attention[b]	Intention Change[c]
Normative Social Influence			
Cognitive Restructuring 1	no	low	wrong
Cognitive Restructuring 2	no	moderate	none
Avoidance/Escape 1	no	high	wrong
Avoidance/Escape 2	no	moderate	right
Avoidance/Escape 3	yes	moderate	none
Self-Esteem 1	no	moderate	wrong
Self-Esteem 2	no	low	none
Self-Esteem 3	no	low	none
Social Activism 1	yes	low	right
Self-Instructional Training 1	yes	moderate	none
Refusal Assertion Learning 1	yes	high	right
Refusal Assertion Practice 1	no	high	right
Ingratiation 1	no	moderate	none
Informational Social Influence			
Prevalence Correction 1	yes	moderate	none
Prevalence Correction 2	yes	moderate	none
Looking Older 1	yes	high	wrong
Looking Older 2	yes	high	right
Adult Modeling	yes	high	wrong
Social Image Model 1	no	low	wrong
Counteradvertising 1	no	moderate	wrong
Counteradvertising 2	yes	moderate	right
Counteradvertising 3	no	high	right
Probing for Information Skills 1	no	moderate	wrong
Polite Debating 1	yes	high	right
Positive Communication 1	yes	low	right
Conversation Initiation 1	yes	low	none
Intimacy 1	yes	low	wrong
Ranking Values 1	no	high	right

continued

"right" change, a 0% to 2% shift indicated no change, and any shift toward increase in curiosity to use indicated a "wrong" change. Numbers after the activity describe modifications and retesting on separate classrooms of promising activities. At least two classrooms were provided with each activity. Project TNT retained activities that showed at least moderate interest and no changes or "right" changes in intention to use tobacco products in the

Table 7.1 Continued

Physical Consequences			
Tobacco Image—Real 1	no	high	right
Tobacco Image—Horrid 1	yes	high	right
Tobacco Image—Horrid 2	no	high	none
Myth Buster 1	yes	high	none
Myth Buster 2	yes	high	right
Listening 1	yes	high	none
Disease Card 1	no	high	right
Court Case 1	no	high	right
Funeral 1	yes	high	right
Funeral 2	yes	high	right
Addiction Role 1	yes	high	wrong
Disease Role 1	yes	high	right
Film on Consequences 1	yes	high	none
Consequences Tree 1	yes	high	none
Bidding 1	yes	high	right

a. Yes = any significant increase in learning.
b. Low = < 40% of sample reported interest in the activity; moderate = 40%-59% reporting interest; high = ≥ 60% reporting interest.
c. Wrong = any change toward increase in curiosity to use; none = < 3% change toward decreased intention to use; right = ≥ 3% change toward decreased intention to use.

future, so that there would be 8 core activities from each of the three types of curricula. The project retained a total of 2 general activities and 24 core activities, or approximately 50% of those tested in the component study phase of development.

One Experimental Component Study Example of Curriculum Development: Refusal Assertion Skills Training

The activity often thought to be central to the social influence approach is refusal assertion training (Del Greco, 1980; Flay et al., 1983; Glynn, 1989). This section describes an example of a component study, conducted separately from those depicted in Table 7.1, that investigated the "active" parts of this activity. Current school-based tobacco use prevention programs with a social-influence orientation emphasize three distinct components in the teaching of refusal assertion skills: (a) providing a list of types of effective refusal assertion strategies, and having students demonstrate each strategy; (b) requiring students to practice saying "no" in the classroom, either using strategies from this list or generating their own; and (c) coaching students to perform the role-play behavior well and providing social reinforcement when students demonstrate good use of these skills in the classroom (i.e., motivating good performance). These components usually are provided in one or two 45-minute lessons to classrooms of approximately 30 students (e.g., Flay, 1985; Flay et al., 1985, 1988; Hansen, Johnson, et al., 1988; Silvestri & Flay, 1989).

The type of refusal assertion training activity that would be most helpful to youth depends on what mediates the refusal skill deficit; that is, the most appropriate instruction is contingent on whether the deficit is knowledge based or performance based (Bellack & Hersen, 1977; Franco, Chistoff, Crimmins, & Kelly, 1983; Gambrill & Richey, 1975; Kelly, 1982; Sussman, 1989). Teaching refusal assertion strategies would help remedy a learning deficit, whereas promoting practice would help remedy a performance deficit due to anxiety or lack of practice of already learned strategies. Coaching from the teacher to demonstrate good performance may help remedy a motivational performance deficit. Simply to please the teacher, a student may perform a better refusal assertion role play after receiving a "pep talk" that requests improved performance. Improved performance due to a motivational manipulation assumes that the student already has learned and practiced the skill. Possibly, improved performance due to a motivational manipulation could lead to intention change to reconcile the student's attitudes with his or her behavior (e.g., to reduce cognitive dissonance; Eiser, 1980). We attempted to ascertain whether refusal assertion skills deficits could be improved through conditions that (a) teach ways to say "no," (b) have students practice saying "no," or (c) try to motivate students to say "no" effectively through use of a counterattitudinal advocacy procedure and teacher praise for improved performance (Turner et al., 1993).

Refusal self-efficacy, assertiveness of refusal assertion strategies used, and behavioral intentions are the major immediate outcome variables in refusal assertion role-play studies (e.g., Graham et al., 1989; Rohrbach, Graham, Hansen, Flay, & Johnson, 1987). Conceptually, an effective refusal assertion curriculum should increase one's refusal self-efficacy (subjective ability to refuse tobacco offers), increase the assertiveness of the refusal assertion strategies one uses during a role play and the way one performs these strategies, and possibly decrease one's behavioral intention to use tobacco in the future. Because behavioral intention is among the best psychosocial predictors of future tobacco use (Fishbein, 1982), it often is considered the most important measure of the effectiveness of a curriculum component.

One class from each of four schools in southern California was randomly selected to participate in the study (one rural and one urban junior high school, and one rural and one urban high school). A randomized, three-group, within-and-between-subjects design was used to determine which of the educational strategies was most effective in improving refusal assertion performance. Students *within* each of the four classes were randomly assigned to one of the three conditions—Learning, Practice, or Motivation (i.e., there was an individual level of assignment to conditions).

Students were removed from class individually and asked to participate in the study. Accompanying the student in a separate classroom were an adult female facilitator (teacher) and an adult female rater. After completing a brief written pretest, each student participated in a refusal assertion role-play pretest that involved up to seven repetitions of refusal assertion responses to the same scenario (i.e., in response to an offer of a cigarette made by the facilitator) in order to carefully tap students' maximum pretest skill level. Each pretest role play was assessed by a rater and the facilitator. Next, the rater left the room and the facilitator delivered one of three 30-minute instructional conditions to the student. The student was told in each condition that the activity could apply to cigarettes or to smokeless tobacco. In the Knowledge condition the student was taught 10 types of responses in an iterative process, without practicing these responses in any role-play situations. In the Practice condition, specific refusal strategies were not taught to the student; rather, the student practiced how to say "no" in 16 different role-played social contexts provided by the adult facilitator, without feedback. The Motivation condition involved the use of a counterattitudinal advocacy manipulation in which the facilitator discussed the importance of maintaining a positive attitude and demonstrating that one can do the task well. Self-affirmations to do the task well were elicited from the student and realistic-sounding student responses to a role-played tobacco offer were rewarded with positive verbal feedback. After the instructional condition was provided, the rater returned to the room and the student completed a posttest questionnaire and engaged in the refusal assertion role play, using the same scenario as in the pretest role play.

This three-condition true field experimental component study of the differential effects of these three components yielded improvement in role-played behavioral skill to refuse tobacco offers that was evident in both the Knowledge and the Practice conditions but not in the Motivation condition. In these same two conditions, skills training also led to a significant decrease in students' intention to use smokeless tobacco in the future but not cigarettes. It is unclear why students' intention to use smokeless tobacco decreased significantly, whereas their intention to use cigarettes did not change. Perhaps students have received much more information prior to this study about the undesirability of smoking than about smokeless tobacco use. Prevention of smokeless tobacco use is a relatively recent phenomenon (Sussman, 1989); awareness that smokeless tobacco is a product one should refuse could have led to a change in intention to use that product. A focus on engaging students in Knowledge and Practice components of refusal assertion training appears warranted.

TESTING OF FULL CURRICULUM: INTEGRATING ACTIVITIES, FEASIBILITY, AND PILOT STUDIES

After theoretical refinements and additional assessments are completed, alternative activities are contrasted, and relatively efficacious activities are retained, (a) the activities must be combined in some sequence within a single lesson, (b) lessons must be combined in some sequence within a single curriculum, (c) the workability (i.e., feasibility) of the whole curriculum should be established, and (d) the whole curriculum should be pilot tested before going to a field trial stage.

Combining Activities

Due to classroom time limitations, previous successfully applied curricula have been able to include approximately four activities in a lesson, when designed for an approximately 45-minute classroom period (e.g., Botvin & Eng, 1979; Flay et al., 1988; Hansen, Graham, et al., 1988). The first activity is a review or a summary of the previous material or an introduction to what will be discussed that day. The second and third activities present new substantive material to the class. These may be substantively independent activities, in which case the order usually is arbitrary. Alternatively, one activity may build on the other, and go second. The final activity summarizes the new material and introduces any homework activities.

Of course, some flexibility needs to be built into the construction of a lesson because of the myriad school variables that necessitate variations in implementation. For example, class periods vary greatly in length, from approximately 35 to 55 minutes. Thus the researcher and health educator should identify core versus optional material within a lesson. As a workable possibility, the final review activity could be considered optional (Sussman, Galaif, et al., 1989).

Combining Lessons

Curriculum lesson sequence should allow for repetition, and gradual mastery of material and attitude change, in keeping with the health education literature and basic learning research (Anderson & Creswell, 1976; Atkins, 1978; Flay et al., 1988). In other words, lessons should be imparted in a "building block" fashion: (a) first lessons introduce the curriculum content to the students, focus on improving student listening skills, and try to enhance student interest in the material; (b) lessons that impart general knowledge and goals are taught before providing specific facts; (c) lessons that impart skills knowledge are taught before lessons that encourage practice of that material; and (d) final lessons summarize the material, prime the students to remember the material, and encourage some type of public commitment to not engage in the risk behavior.

Even with adherence to this "building block" principle, a variety of lesson orders are possible. One way of establishing order preference is through independent judgments of health educators. However, order preference showed little consistency across four health educator judges when this task was attempted for Project TNT (average Kendall's coefficient of concordance = .21 across 10 lessons and four curricula). Student-generated order preferences, or studies that systematically vary curriculum order and assess immediate impact, might result in a more appropriate determination. However, these later tasks would demand the undertaking of numerous additional studies that might not be imperative to the whole process. Thus in Project TNT, lessons were combined using a prespecified protocol to be used across curricula. An introductory lesson would be followed by cognitive-perspective-related lessons, then behavioral (role-playing) lessons, then decision-making-related and activism lessons, and finally a public commitment lesson.

It is important for the researcher to identify key lessons that should be taught intact (ones that have shown a relatively strong impact on mediators of change) because a curriculum may be modified during some future implementation so as to better blend in with specific school characteristics. For example, lesson plans may be blended in with material from a course other than health, in which case some integration of a content area (e.g., English) with the health area would be entertained (Holcomb et al., 1984). In addition, teachers may not have the time to implement a complete "canned" curriculum as planned (e.g., 10 lessons over 2 weeks), due to planning time, school class length, and schedule (Tricker & Davis, 1988). Although a curriculum can be spread out a little (e.g., from 2 weeks to 3 weeks) in delivery, deletion of material may render a previously successful curriculum ineffective.

A draft version of a curriculum should be written, adhering to the "building block" principle (i.e., each lesson logically flows from the last lesson) and key lessons should be highlighted. After the whole curriculum is pieced together, the researcher should engage in feasibility and pilot studies. Feasibility studies help determine whether a chosen sequence works at all with students without doing an extensive amount of data collection. Pilot studies are needed to get a detailed assessment of curriculum implementation and immediate impact.

Feasibility Studies

Feasibility studies involve the classroom delivery of full draft lessons to get subjective judgments of their workability. To maximize the usefulness of this procedure, at least two judges should be present in the class (e.g., the project health educator and a project observer) to provide independent judgments of the quality of program delivery (e.g., Hansen, Graham, et al., 1988). The effectiveness of the lesson is determined by (a) obvious considerations such as length of lesson and class participation, and (b) health educator and classroom observer judgments of students' reactions to the lesson while it is being delivered. The emphasis of this qualitative evaluation approach is on process—how events happen and the possible meanings of events (McLaughlin & Owen, 1987).

Strengths and Weaknesses

The strength of this approach is that multiple activities can be provided together and gross evaluations of the whole package can be made by health educators and observers under "real-world" conditions. Thus issues such as lesson duration, workability of current lesson sequence, and continued student involvement can be addressed fruitfully. The weakness of this approach is that "soft" data are collected that may be subject to experimenter bias. Collection of posttest-only data from students and use of multiple observers (e.g., calculation of interrater agreement on scales rated by the health educator and observer) can be accomplished to partially alleviate this difficulty. After one or two feasibility trials, the researcher should have identified the rough edges in the curriculum and refined the curriculum to a more workable form. Additional feasibility tests, if needed, are completed as part of the pilot study phase of Step 4.

Application to Project TNT

The main information gathered here was that the presentation of some information was taking too much time, particularly in Lesson 1 (the introductory lesson) in each curriculum. We also learned that there were some difficulties with extensive review periods related to a TNT game and a few curriculum-specific lessons. For example, it became clear that debating was a learning deficit among 7th graders and that it would take two lessons, not one, to teach this skill. It was replaced with social problem solving in the informational social influence curriculum. Again, lecturing for any length of time was not an effective means of instruction. We did achieve what appeared to be theoretically sound curricula; any rating of discussion content would reveal a good check on the manipulations completed.

Pilot Studies

Pilot studies are the testing of a near-final-draft, whole curriculum, involving one-group or between-groups pretest-posttest designs with a small number of units (classes, schools) per condition. A variety of pilot study designs are possible. For example, in Project TVSFP, a school-based mass-media-enhanced cigarette and drug use prevention project conducted in southern California, one pilot study was accomplished that involved providing two different curricula to 7th graders at two "matched" schools (one curriculum per school; Flay et al., 1988). Student pretest and posttest self-report questionnaires, and health educator (curriculum teacher), classroom observer (the classroom teacher), principal, and parent posttest-only self-report questionnaires were collected, as were daily homework completion rates and health educator, observer, and student daily process ratings of lessons.

Strengths and Weaknesses

The strengths of this approach are that a thorough implementation and immediate impact evaluation can be accomplished and field trial evaluation materials can be drafted and finalized. On the other hand, pilot studies are a relatively expensive means of evaluation; thus only a few replications usually can be completed. This limits the generalizability of the findings and possibilities for further curriculum improvements. The usefulness of a pilot study is contingent, in part, on there having been careful work done prior to this last step of curriculum development.

The curriculum is ready for a formal test when (a) it consists of activities developed through empirical means to counteract key acquisition variables; (b) these activities are of reasonable time length, relatively high in interest, and relatively high in perceived helpfulness; (c) activities and full lessons are placed in a sequence so as to facilitate gradual building of knowledge and lead to desired attitude change; and (d) the whole curriculum has been found to alter theoretical mediators of change (i.e., knowledge, beliefs, attitudes) that, in time, should exert a preventive effect on risk behavior. Manipulation of behavioral intentions to not engage in the risk behavior in the future is desirable, but more difficult to achieve (Flay, 1981; Sussman, Galaif, et al., 1989).

Application to Project TNT

In Project TNT, the pilot study was designed as follows. Each curriculum was delivered to half of the classrooms at a school. A second curriculum was delivered to the other classrooms at the school. The physical consequences and normative social influence curricula were run at the same school; the informational social influence and combined condition curricula were run at a second school. Data collected included workbooks, homework, and student pretest and posttest, teacher-observer, health educator, and principal assessments. Brief focus groups and part of the review sessions were used to ensure theoretical soundness of each curriculum. No contamination across curricula was observed over this 2-week period. All four curricula were revised and then were run again at two more schools. To summarize the pilot study results, "a lot of information had been collected." We knew that we had too much material in the curricula, particularly in the informational social influence and combined influences curricula. Even though we had accomplished a great deal of piloting, additional revisions were made.

In the normative social influence curriculum, a stress-coping activity was revised. Keeping it linked to peer pressure was emphasized. Five minutes were removed from some lessons.

In the informational social influence curriculum, some agreement about terminology still needed working out (scanning, probing, social fact, social image, social awareness). This curriculum had a lot of good material in it and it was theoretically sound (a very difficult task). Unfortunately, it had too much complex material. We deleted a lesson that attempted to counteract adult influences on tobacco use. For example, this lesson instructed students that most adult tobacco users want to quit but have trouble doing it; therefore they don't want their children to start. It may appear that adults are saying, "Do as I say, not as I do," but they really are trying to keep young persons from suffering the pains of addiction. Our students found this material too complex. We could not successfully teach it in one lesson. Also, we modified a new social-problem-solving lesson to make it more focused on assertive behavior. A self-esteem lesson still needed simplification. We decided to define self-esteem as "trusting oneself" and linked it with making independent decisions. "Probing," "scanning," and "intimacy" communication skills were combined. They were instructed as an "effective communication" lesson, using a more strict behavioral format, including the elements of demonstration, modeling, behavioral rehearsal, and feedback and social reinforcement.

In the physical consequences curriculum, we needed to simplify instruction of the addiction processes in the role plays and otherwise. We did this by having students read cards and briefly act out what they had read, rather than having students try to rehearse and perform complex disease role playing. The bidding activity (which attacked the cost of tobacco use) was made brief so that we could make more of the use of a disease probability card activity, which provided information on relative probability of consequences.

In the combined condition, there was just too much material. Generally, 5 minutes of material was shaved off all lessons.

EIGHT

Lesson Contents and Implementation

This chapter presents the real "nitty-gritty" of delivery of the prevention component of Project TNT: the lesson contents, classroom management issues and solutions, composition of the Project TNT questionnaire, and the data collection procedure. In other words, the pragmatics of the health education and data collection activities are presented in detail.

CURRICULA CONTENTS

The four curricula (see Appendices A to E) contain similar motivational and commitment elements in Lessons 1, 9, and 10. Also, each curriculum includes unique material that confronts either (a) normative social influence (Abrams, Selski, Craig, Barovich, & Sussman, 1989), (b) informational social influence (Barovich, Craig, Selski, Abrams, & Sussman, 1989), (c) physical consequences (Hahn et al., 1989), or (d) combined normative and informational social influences plus physical consequences (Selski, Craig, Barovich, & Sussman, 1989). The contents of these curricula are described next.

Commonalities

In all four curricula, Lesson 1 involves a participatory listening exercise (the "Telephone Game") to engage the students in the curriculum and motivate them to pay attention to the subsequent material. Also, in the first lesson, students are introduced to a major reason youth engage in tobacco use and are provided with tobacco product information. The reason for using tobacco described to the students is tied to the content of the particular curriculum. Finally, students are introduced to the "TNT Game," a competitive team game used to help maintain student involvement and maximize homework return rate. The winning team, consisting of about five participants per class (usually six teams per class), wins a prize such as a food coupon (donated by a community food establishment) worth $2 per student.

In all four curricula, Lessons 9 and 10 overlap in content. The 9th lesson teaches students to become involved in protesting tobacco use by writing a letter advocating no tobacco use. The content of the letter reflects the rest of the curriculum contents; for example, one will not be liked if one uses tobacco (normative social influence curriculum), tobacco will not provide the social images one might think it does (informational social influence curriculum), tobacco use causes negative physical consequences (physical consequences curriculum), or all three messages (in the combined condition). During the 10th lesson, a video is filmed in the classroom, using a TV news program format, in which students summarize what they have learned in the project and share a commitment they have made about tobacco use—that is, to teach someone what they have learned about tobacco use or to not start use themselves. The students view the video they developed at the end of the same class period.

Finally, in all four curricula, both major forms of tobacco used by youth are addressed, and are addressed in the same proportions across curricula. Specifically, 20% of the language referring to tobacco products mentions smokeless tobacco, 5% refers to pipes or cigars, 10% refers to the generic term *tobacco*, and 65% refers to cigarette smoking in each curriculum. Thus any differential effects on future cigarette versus smokeless tobacco use behavior would not be due to the tobacco product focus of a curriculum.

Normative Social Influence Curriculum

In the normative social influence curriculum, Lesson 2, students are introduced to aspects of peer pressure and peer group acceptance. Resistance to peer pressure to use tobacco is discussed, and the students learn that they can still be liked by their friends (if they refuse peer group tobacco offers) because they serve multiple functions within their groups ("ingratiation"). In Lesson 3, students are introduced to a thought-changing process ("cognitive restructuring") that, through use of "thought bubbles," teaches them that situations are often less threatening than they initially appear. In particular, they learn that they may be respected by their friends for refusing tobacco offers. In Lesson 4, students learn the importance of being assertive in peer pressure situations and are introduced to the various ways of saying "no" to tobacco offers. In Lesson 5, students are introduced to the "KAT" decision-making process (know the problem, know the alternatives, think the problem through) as a means of avoiding tobacco use pressure situations. In Lesson 6, students view a videotape depicting ways to say "no," and then they practice the methods they have learned through role plays, practiced in groups and performed in front of the class. In Lesson 7, students continue to practice methods of saying "no." Finally, in Lesson 8, students practice escape techniques (from tobacco use situations) and then are introduced to stress reduction techniques that they can use to keep themselves calm in peer pressure situations.

Informational Social Influence Curriculum

In the informational social influence curriculum, in Lesson 2, students compare the assumed prevalence of tobacco use in their class with actual use to reduce overestimation errors. In Lesson 3, students discuss ways to achieve social images they desire without using tobacco. Also, students participate in a "restructuring" activity, in which they indicate whether they "agree" or "disagree" with various statements by standing under signs. In this procedure, students learn that most students do not believe that social images sometimes associated with tobacco use are true (e.g., that tobacco use makes someone look older). In Lesson 4, students discuss the entertainment and advertisement media's social images of tobacco use that might influence individuals to use tobacco. A videotape is shown that corrects inaccurate social image depictions of tobacco use. In Lesson 5, students practice techniques to improve their self-esteem: for example, by being prompted to acknowledge their own positive characteristics. In Lesson 6, students learn to identify key aspects of effective communication and practice communication skills in role-play situations. They are instructed that by learning effective communication skills they can acquire more accurate information about social events. In Lesson 7, students practice how to develop open-ended questions as a means of enhancing their conversational skills. Finally, in Lesson 8, students learn a method of decision making to help them make the best choices in difficult interpersonal situations (e.g., how to speak with a friend who has not returned a belonging that was borrowed).

Physical Consequences Curriculum

In the physical consequences curriculum, in Lesson 2, students are introduced to physical consequences of tobacco use and learn decision-making skills specifically dealing with consequences. In Lesson 3, students learn about the course of tobacco use addiction through use of role-play demonstrations of different stages of tobacco experimentation (first trial, tolerance and enjoyment, addiction, health problems). In Lesson 4, students discuss in detail tobacco-related diseases and role-play disease symptoms. In Lesson 5, students calculate the financial costs of addiction to tobacco products and identify facts about tobacco use consequences through playing a team game ("prevention baseball"). In Lesson 6, students practice horrific imagery to provide a memory association of tobacco use to negative physical consequences in situations where they are likely to use it. In Lesson 7, students discuss the death of Sean Marsee, a high school track star who was a heavy user of smokeless tobacco. They also begin preparation of a class presentation about tobacco use consequences, which they perform in Lesson 10. Finally, in Lesson 8, students identify the relative risks of tobacco-use-related diseases, comparing those who use tobacco to nonusers.

Combined Curriculum

In the combined curriculum, in Lesson 1, students learn to correct inflated prevalence estimates of tobacco use, as well as learn multiple reasons for tobacco use and other material common across curricula. In Lesson 2, students learn about the course of tobacco addiction and disease through use of role plays and identify the physical and social consequences associated with tobacco use. In Lesson 3, students practice techniques to improve their self-esteem, including being prompted to acknowledge their own positive characteristics. In Lesson 4, students are introduced to peer pressure, and they discuss how they can resist peer pressure to use tobacco and still be accepted for their other attributes by those who offer them tobacco. In addition, students are taught about "thought-changing" processes in order to learn that they may be respected by friends for refusing a tobacco offer. In Lesson 5, students are introduced to the importance of effective communication. They practice effective listening skills, initiating conversations, and developing open-ended questions. In Lesson 6, students learn the importance of being assertive and are introduced to various ways of saying "no." In Lesson 7, students view the videotape depicting the different ways to say "no," and then they practice these methods. Finally, in Lesson 8, students discuss the ways in which the media portray tobacco-related "social images" that influence individuals to use tobacco. Students view a videotape that corrects false social images about tobacco use depicted by the public media. Thus in Lessons 2 through 8, the combined condition is composed of three lessons of normative social influence curriculum material, three lessons of informational social influence curriculum material, and one lesson of physical consequences curriculum material.

In summary, curricula were developed to counteract these three causes of tobacco use. Each of the three curricula was developed to counteract a single general-component cause of tobacco use: (a) normative social influence, (b) informational social influence, or (c) physical consequences. The fourth curriculum combined all three prevention components. Many of the types of activities (e.g. role playing) overlapped across curricula, but the information content was unique to a particular curriculum.

CLASSROOM MANAGEMENT

This next section describes classroom management problems and solutions. Good classroom management is the sine qua non of implementation. Thus we provide some useful tips here. The "keys to good classroom management" are presented in outline form to be of maximum immediate usefulness to the health educator as a proactive guide to planning instruction of the curriculum.

Types of Management Difficulties and Solutions

The types of management techniques that are likely to be successful depend, of course, on the nature of the classroom behavior problem. There are at least five roots of behavior difficulties: (a) academic frustration, (b) confusion and limit testing, (c) impulsiveness, (d) rebellion, and (e) group processes.

Academic frustration (e.g., angry or restless behavior, cheating) refers to the difficulties stemming from a student's inability to participate in the class because he or she is unable to grasp the material as presented. Keeping material simple, individualizing instruction in a programmed instruction format (e.g., in steps; shaping and tailoring), or using multiple learning channels (i.e., kinds of materials used; materials that require seeing, hearing, touching, smelling, and behaving) can help control this difficulty.

Confusion and limit testing (e.g., provocative behavior) refers to difficulties stemming from a student's being unsure what the classroom rules are, as he or she can often be when provided with substitute teachers, when beginning a new course, or when beginning a new topic within a course. Making rules explicit, making consequences such as point systems explicit, and clearly and positively introducing the subject matter can help control this difficulty. Also, humor can help.

Impulsiveness (e.g., bumping into other students, speaking out of turn) refers to the difficulties stemming from a student's not thinking before he or she acts. Providing self-instructions while teaching material (e.g., stop signs) or "soft reprimands" (reprimands only audible to the student) can help control this difficulty.

Rebellion (e.g., defiant behavior) refers to the difficulties stemming from a student's trying to define the limits of his or her own behavior without input from others. Making the points that others in the class receive contingent on this person's behavior, praising cooperative behavior on this person's part, sometimes loud reprimands, or enlisting this person's support to control others (paradoxical intention) can help control this difficulty.

Group processes (e.g., subgrouping, class norms versus the new teacher, changes in class composition) refers to the difficulties stemming from competition within the class or from changes placed on an existing class. To help control this difficulty, some limit-testing strategies are relevant; so are changing seating arrangements, creating randomly organized class groups, and manipulating cohesiveness within the class (e.g., accomplishing a task that takes the effort of all members; see Hetherington & Parke, 1975, pp. 455-461; O'Leary & Wilson, 1975, chap. 7).

Keys to Good Classroom Management[1]

I. Preparation
   A. Plan classroom procedures and rules in detail.
   B. Initial contact is very important—you never get a second chance to make a good first impression.
   C. Know your material.
   D. Begin immediately to establish your credibility and leadership in the classroom.
   E. Be professional—look professional.

II. Clearly Define Your Expectations of the Class
   A. Have clear ideas about behavior you expect.
      Decide what minor inappropriate behavior can be ignored.
   B. Let students know what types of behavior are and are not acceptable. Tell students:
      Pay attention
      Do not make judgments or put-downs of others.
      Be respectful of each other.
      Know your material.
      Raise your hand and wait until you are called upon.
      Talk one at a time during class discussion.
   C. Explain to the students how you plan on handling discipline.
      Rules must be consistent and clear.
      Only one warning will be given before consequences are applied.
      Include positive consequences for good behavior as well as negative consequences for inappropriate behavior.
III. Monitor the Class Throughout the Presentation
   A. Stand or sit where you can see and be seen by all the students during the period.
   B. Walk around the room.
   C. Praise students for good behavior.
   D. Use classroom structure.
      Desk arrangement
      Student grouping
      Use space effectively
IV. Stop Inappropriate Behavior Quickly
   A. Walk up to the student's desk (at times this is enough to stop the inappropriate behavior).
   B. Maintain eye contact until the behavior stops. If the behavior continues:
   C. Ask the student to state the rule he or she has broken.
   D. Tell the student what you expect him or her to be doing.
   E. Give the student a chance to change seats if he or she feels tempted to misbehave.
   F. Tell the student to stop inappropriate behavior and explain consequence.
   G. *Follow through consistently.*

A teacher can use several classroom management techniques to help facilitate positive learning. The methods used will depend a lot on the physical structure (atmosphere) of the classroom as well as the energy level of the individual students. A positive, nurturing attitude maintained by the teacher will help promote a positive class experience. For example, it helps to hold the attitude that each student is unique and worthwhile to the class. This will help in dealing with the varied issues and problems that may arise in a classroom. Consistency is crucial in order for teacher and student to have a positive relationship. When the class is aware of what is expected of them, and rules are consistently enforced, the classroom experience for all individuals involved is a favorable one.

QUESTIONNAIRE DEVELOPMENT AND CONTENTS

Questionnaire Development

Project TNT questionnaire development in part relied on a long history of questionnaires developed at the institute that had already established internal consistency, test-retest reliability, and concurrent and predictive validity of many of the behavioral and psychosocial measures used in this study (e.g., Collins et al., 1987; Graham, Flay, Johnson, Hansen, Grossman, & Sobel, 1984; Graham et al., 1985; MacKinnon et al., 1991; Sussman, Flay, et al., 1986). Also, a general protocol of development/refinement was followed.

First, a thorough search of the literature and other questionnaires was made before selecting questionnaire items for the student questionnaire. Next, a draft version questionnaire was developed and delivered to groups of approximately 250 7th-grade students from four junior high schools in southern California (total $N = 1,000$). A total of six health educators and 12 teacher-observers helped complete and refine implementation and process measures. Also, our health educators worked closely with the research staff to develop and refine curricula knowledge items.

Item selection for the main student questionnaire was determined by the necessity for including (a) proximal aspects of the program (e.g., participation in, knowledge of, and attitudes toward material presented—"implementation and process items"); (b) tobacco-use-"sensitive" aspects of the program (e.g., items correlated with smoking and smokeless tobacco use intentions and behaviors); and (c) aspects that might mediate program response (e.g., baseline program expectancies). When developing or choosing items that might mediate program response, we had to attend to several criteria, including: (a) at least two items for each construct had to be tapped if at all possible; (b) the items chosen for each construct had to show moderately significant intercorrelations (i.e., r = at least .25); (c) items had to show good response variability (i.e., the rule of thumb used for most attitude items was that at least 10% of sample had to respond in each category to show sufficient response variability to use the item in the main study); and (d) items chosen had to be understandable to the students (all students' questions about different items, and percentages of students completing each item, were recorded). Regarding the implementation or process items, criteria for selection included: (a) items had to be closely anchored to material imparted in the program; and (b) items had to be clearly understandable to the students, teacher-observers, or health educators. A standard-vocabulary-level list was used to tailor words used on the final questionnaires. A 5th-grade reading level was established as a ceiling on most words used for this 7th-grade audience. One further decision rule in Project TNT was to decrease the number of response categories on many of the psychosocial items (e.g., from ratings scales to binary responses) so that these items could be more easily completed by young adolescents and more items could be completed.

Questionnaire Contents in Main Student Surveys

Questionnaire contents in the 20-page large-scale Project TNT surveys were composed of four sections. The first or *core section* was always placed at the front of the questionnaire, after the cover page. The remaining three sections contained different internally consistent sets of items, and they were rotated in order to produce three questionnaire forms (ABC, BCA, and CAB orders). Core items included ethnic group, living situation, trial and current use of smokeless tobacco, trial and current use of cigarettes, trial and current use of alcohol, and intention to use these substances in the future. Also included were social influence self-efficacy items (Stacy et al., 1992), social desirability items (Crowne & Marlowe, 1960), and classroom climate items (a total of 48 items).

Four behavioral outcome measures were derived from the core section: "Have you ever tried cigarettes?" ("yes" or "no"); "Have you ever tried smokeless tobacco?" ("yes" or "no"); "How often do you smoke cigarettes?" ("a few times each month" or greater was coded as weekly use); and "How often do you use smokeless tobacco?" ("a few times each month" or greater was coded as weekly use). Forms of smokeless tobacco were described on the cover page of the questionnaire, which was reviewed for the class by the data collector. Students were instructed to code chewing tobacco and snuff as both being forms of smokeless tobacco.

In a *social section* of the questionnaire, items measured positive or negative reactions to others' tobacco use, latch-key-related items (Richardson et al., 1989), tobacco and alcohol use prevalence items (e.g., Sussman, Dent, Mestel-Rauch, et al., 1988), peer and family tobacco use and approval of subject's use of tobacco products (e.g., MacKinnon et al., 1991), peer commitment (e.g., Sussman, Dent, Simon, et al., 1993), family conflict, school and nonschool activity participation, and group self-identification (e.g., Sussman et al., 1990; Sussman, Dent, McAdams, et al., 1994). There were a total of 42 items in this section of the questionnaire.

A *knowledge section* of the questionnaire included items that measured manipulations within the normative social influence, informational social influence, and physical consequences conditions (as discussed below). Approximately two items had been developed from Lessons 2 through 8 of each curriculum (Sussman, Dent, Stacy, Hodgson, et al., 1993). In addition, this section contained school prevention expectancy items (e.g., Sussman, Dent, Brannon, et al., 1989), tobacco use outcome expectancy items (e.g., Stacy, Dent, et al., 1990), and school tobacco policy items. A total of 78 items were in this section. Even though there were a greater number of items in this section than the others, the number of response choices per item (e.g., presence of checklist items) was far fewer.

A total of 45 *knowledge items* tapped learning of the three separate prevention components. Each knowledge item was multiple choice and provided two to three wrong answers along with one correct answer. Approximately two items tapped material from Lesson 2 through 8 in each component. For example, normative social influence knowledge items with their correct answers included Q: "You will be liked more by a friend if"—A: "you agree with most of their opinions but not all of them" (Lesson 2) and Q: "Which of the following is reversing the pressure? saying"—A: "'I don't smoke and you shouldn't either'" (Lesson 6). Informational social influence knowledge items with their correct answers included Q: "Most 7th-grade students agree that smoking cigarettes makes young people"—A: "none of the above" (i.e., not look older, not look glamorous; Lesson 4) and Q: "Which of the following is the best example of an open-ended question"—A: "'What did you think about yesterday's class?'" (the other choices are questions that do not facilitate extended responses; Lesson 7). Physical consequences knowledge items with their correct answers included Q: "Nicotine withdrawal means"—A: "a person will feel bad if they cannot get any tobacco" (Lesson 3) and Q: "Who is Sean Marsee?"—A: "a teenager who died from tobacco use" (Lesson 7).

Finally, the *personal section* of the questionnaire contained items on risk taking (Collins et al., 1987), self-esteem (Rosenberg, 1972), coping effort to not use tobacco (Sussman, Brannon, et al., 1993), perceived stress (Cohen, Kamarck, & Mermelstein, 1983), loneliness, attitude toward tobacco use, assertiveness (Gambrill & Richey, 1978), health risk factors (Sussman, Dent, Simon, et al., 1993; Sussman, Dent, Stacy, et al., in press), orientation toward "wellness," past-future orientation, and self-rated physical attractiveness (Sussman, Dent, Stacy, et al., in press). This section was composed of 52 items.

An *addendum* contained six parental socioeconomic status items, three regarding each parent (job name as a fill-in-the-blank item, job type, educational attainment). A final section tapped process ratings of the Project TNT curriculum delivered, as discussed below.

The 1-year and 2-year follow-up questionnaires prompted the subjects' memory concerning their use of cigarettes, smokeless tobacco, alcohol, or marijuana the prior year and then prompted recall of curriculum contents and requested process ratings in a final series of 14 items. The 1- and 2-year follow-up questionnaire increased in length slightly by adding violent event items (Sussman, Dent, et al., 1994) and marijuana behavior items, although the number of knowledge items was reduced by around 15%. Our previous research suggests that 80% to 90% of a large sample of students in one class period can complete approximately 90 items in 7th grade, 105 items in 8th grade, 120 to 140 items in 9th grade, 140 to 170 items in 10th grade, and 200 or more items by 11th grade.

Student Program Evaluation Items

The program evaluation portion of the immediate posttest questionnaire included 21 process evaluation adjective items (on 3-point scales written as *yes, somewhat,* and *no* or *not really,* on the first page) and nine implementation or process evaluation items (on 3- to 6-point scales, on the second page). On the first page, students were instructed to "take a minute to think about the last 2 weeks of this class. Think about the topics and activities done each day. Think about all 10 lessons, and then try to form a general opinion about the class. Overall, did you find the class topics and activities . . . acceptable, believable, [etc.]?" The adjective items were all process-type. The items were analyzed as an index consisting of the mean of all items. Also, four of the items from this index were analyzed individually (class control/acceptability, program effectiveness/helpfulness, program understandability, and teaching effectiveness/organization) to permit a comparison of students' process ratings with those of the health educators and teacher-observers. On the second page, students were instructed that "some classes have just finished a 10-day program with Project TNT. We would like to know how students feel about the program." Then they were requested to complete the nine items if they were in a Project TNT program condition. These items included an assessment of the number of homework assignments completed, program usefulness, and whether the students would recommend that other students the same age be administered this program. The only implementation item assessed of students was the number of homework assignments returned to the health educator.

Abbreviated Student Surveys

It should be mentioned that for individually tracked students who could not be surveyed in the classroom, *abbreviated surveys* were administered by telephone. Students phoned at home received abbreviated 20-minute surveys that requested core information including identifying data (e.g., highest grade level achieved, birthdate, previous school attendance), tobacco and alcohol use behavior and intentions, demographic variables (e.g., current living situation, current language spoken at home), peer approval for tobacco use, knowledge items, and an open-ended student comments item (approximately a total of 40 items). The numbers and types of items varied by year of the survey, but these questionnaires enabled calculation of behavior outcomes and provided some means of obtaining manipulation check data.

Role-Play Assessments

Data on refusal assertion and conversational skill role playing were collected (Sussman, Stacy, et al., 1993). The contents of the refusal assertion assessments were described in Chapter 7 as a refusal assertion training component study. The conversational skills assessment involved a scenario dealing with initiating a conversation with a peer who was in an apparently compromising situation (locked out of the house). The assessment instruments used were of the same type as the assertion refusal instrument (see Sussman, Stacy, et al., 1993).

Health Educator and Teacher-Observer Program Evaluation Items at Immediate Posttest

Health Educators

Health educators completed three types of ratings of curriculum implementation and process. One type of rating was an

11-item lesson evaluation that was completed after each class taught (mostly on 7-point rating scales; e.g., "How enthusiastic was the class during this session?" rated from *unenthusiastic* [1] to *enthusiastic* [7]). They also completed a 13-item end-of-program evaluation, one for each class group taught (completed after Lesson 10, mostly on 4-point rating scales; e.g., "How effective do you think this curriculum is in preventing tobacco use?" rated from *very ineffective* [a] to *very effective* [d]). Finally, they completed a 13-item overall curriculum evaluation at the end of the school year that assessed four items for each curriculum (mostly on 4-point rating scales). The curriculum evaluation also included a ranking item of relative perceived effectiveness of curricula. In addition, health educators kept records of each of their students' attendance and homework returns.

Regarding implementation measurement, delivery fidelity items were asked solely of health educators. These items are described measuring gross to subtle disruptions in implementation (see Chapter 9). Adherence (was the curriculum delivered at all) was not measured through any questionnaire item because all other items depended on whether a curriculum was delivered at all. Exposure (how much of the curriculum was delivered) was measured through use of open-ended responses to the items "activity omitted" and "activity not completed," contained on the lesson evaluation form. Reinvention (was the curriculum changed in delivery even though all lessons were delivered) was a binary item from the lesson evaluation composed of the average of responses completed by a health educator across lessons; it read, "Was the session taught *as written?*" ("yes" or "no"). Finally, the smoothness of delivery item also was from the lesson evaluation form and read, "Did the session proceed smoothly?" ("yes" or "no").

Teacher-Observers

Teacher-observers completed a nine-page school staff survey consisting of 19 evaluation items (on 4- to 5-point rating scales) that was administered at immediate posttest. For example, Item 7 read, "How effective do you think the TNT curriculum will be in teaching this age group of students to resist drugs (including tobacco)?" Responses ranged from *very ineffective* (a) to *very effective* (d). Anonymity of responses was assured.

DATA COLLECTION[2]

Data collection involves several steps that often are not presented explicitly in published manuscripts (see Custer et al., 1989). Consent was already discussed in Chapter 5. Other data collection tasks are described below.

Creating a Database

A database is the broad file of information from which all reports are drawn. A PC file computer program was used. A separate database for each school was used in light of the volume of information required. For our purposes, the only schools requiring individual student files were the actively consented schools, which were the portion of the individual cohort to be tracked.

Student information was obtained through the use of data cards that provided the student's name, sex, date of birth, address, phone number, and parents' names. This information was used to establish all of the student files in each school's database. This core information was updated as it changed, and was the starting point for tracking students throughout the study.

The timing of data card completion depended on the initial consent distribution and school policies. In most cases, cards were distributed at the same time as consents. Teachers were asked to use a few minutes of class time to permit TNT staff members to distribute these materials and have the students complete the information on the data cards. Usually this information was completed by the students in the classroom where they were to be measured. Data cards were completed at the same time that a TNT staff member distributed consents in schools when this procedure occurred. Whenever possible, it was advantageous to obtain both a data card and a school list from the school so that they could be compared and the completeness of the student information could be maximized. Many times one source was missing information that could be obtained from the second.

The student information file looked like this:

IC SC:	001 188 007
CONSENT RECD:	Y
LAST NAME:	GOOD
FIRST:	JOHNNY
MID INITIAL:	B
STREET:	333 LINCOLN AVE
CITY:	PASADENA
ZIP:	91101
AREA CODE:	818
PHONE:	5550472
DOB:	030376
SEX:	M
MOTHER:	JOAN
CURR SC CODE:	001
CURR SC NAME:	LINCOLN ELEM
TEACHER:	JOHNSON
TEACHER CODE:	01
PERIOD:	03
BATCH:	8442
MEASURED:	M
TRUANT:	NEVER
NOTES:	NONE

Identification (ID) numbers were usually assigned after the teacher and period had been entered from classroom rosters received from the school. This assured that as many new students as possible received ID numbers before the classroom measure was administered. The ID number contained the school code (three digits), the survey form number the student would receive (1, 2, or 3), the year the student entered the program (two digits), and the student's rank on the school list. Rank was determined by simply numbering the school list alphabetically (three digits).

Once the data card, school directory, and consent information was received, entered, and alphabetized, the *consent calling list* was created. This list pulled up the names, addresses, and phone numbers of the students who did not return a consent. Callers used this list to telephone parents at home to obtain verbal active consent. As previously mentioned, this procedure was used provided that the school district approved the release of student phone numbers. If the numbers were not released, schools sometimes allowed TNT staff to call on school grounds. This same list was used to achieve higher questionnaire completion rates through a telephone survey, which involved an abbreviated survey administered to no-shows (described earlier in this chapter).

Preparation for Classes

Data collection preparation for classes receiving an anonymous measure involved completing the face of batch envelopes (a separate batch envelope identified each classroom), counting out surveys, and including a class and school summary sheet. For classes receiving a confidential measure, class and school summaries, class lists, school lists, CO and saliva sheets, new student and absentee sheets, student and teacher absentee letters, and envelopes were included as data collection forms. Surveys were precoded with assigned student ID numbers, and then these surveys needed to be sorted and included in the correct class batch envelope. CO and saliva materials (tubes for CO collection, swabs and vials for saliva collection) were packaged for each class as needed. Vitalographs, which were used to measure CO levels, required calibration prior to and on the date of collection.

Classroom Procedure

Each period varied in length from 35 to 55 minutes depending on the school schedule. The main components of each collection involved the following: script delivery, survey distribution, data collector ratings, survey completion instructions, breath or saliva samples, completion of batch envelope, new student and absentee lists, class and school summary sheets, and delivery of absentee surveys. Two data collector roles were present, the "speaker" and the "logger." The speaker provided the verbal directions to the class, and the logger kept track of student forms and recorded biochemical data.

After entering the classroom and giving class introductions, the script was delivered and surveys were distributed. In every collection the first half of the script (which introduced the collection and provided consent-related information) was delivered to the class as written. Next, the speaker used the class list to take roll and call participating students forward to collect their survey. This procedure required a great deal of accuracy because the confidential surveys were precoded with ID numbers. The original objective was to have 75% of each class participate in a confidential survey, and this was achieved. As discussed previously, it was necessary to include an anonymous measure as a means of increasing participation (to over 80%).

During survey distribution, data collectors recorded certain types of data. The speaker recorded batch numbers on the face of the survey. The logger recorded ratings on the CO sheet or saliva sheet. The class list was checked as each student was called. If a student was absent the speaker marked a (9) or (AB) beside that student's name on the survey and set it aside for the logger. The CO and saliva sheets were similarly marked by the logger. Students not listed on the class list were compared to the school list to see if they had been consented to participate. If so, the logger gave them an appropriate survey. If not they were asked to complete a data card and were treated as new students.

The remaining script depended on the type of chemical validation used. At this point, the logger rotated assisting students while the speaker gave instructions on completing the face page of the survey, demonstrated how to respond to example questions, answered any questions, and prompted an orderly collection. The timing of the completion of parental occupation questions and additional instruction was left to the discretion of the speaker as to temperament of the class and their personal preference. Similarly, the timing of the saliva sample was piloted at various points in the collection.

Once students began working independently, the logger and speaker collected biochemical measures. The speaker was responsible for answering student questions, as was a third data collector when available. Surveys were collected and counted 5 to 7 minutes prior to the end of the class period.

Project TNT data collection staff completed a class summary noting the general mood of collection and any disruption factors that may have occurred. The Project TNT school data collection coordinator also completed a school summary sheet regarding any extenuating circumstances that may have affected the collection prior to or on the actual measure date. Absentee packets were left on the day of measure for any students that could not participate due to absence. The batch number for that class was written in ink on the originally prepared survey before it was put in an absentee envelope, and the student's name was written in pencil on the outside of the envelope. The students were asked to take approximately 2 weeks to fill out the surveys and were told to erase their names from the outside of the envelopes before returning them to their teachers. Five packets per classroom were prepared prior to the collection date. Each packet contained a student instruction letter explaining how to fill out the survey.

We handled the collection of these surveys in two ways: the first was to inform the teacher that we would be picking them up within 3 weeks after the day we left them; the second was to put postage on each envelope when they were prepared in the office. The second way seemed to work much better because the students could mail the surveys directly instead of returning them to their teachers. This also relieved teachers of extra work. In many cases, we had to resort to phone surveys for collection of confidential data.

Phone Surveys

Youth who were absent from testing in the classroom ("no show" subjects), especially those from the intensively tracked cohort, as well as the out-of-school youth (dropouts or graduates), completed either written self-report questionnaires mailed to their homes (along with stamped self-addressed envelopes) or phone surveys. Response rate to the phone survey method was high after acquisition of phone numbers (over 80%).

Data Collection Lists

Several types of lists were kept, the *phone calling list* described above, a school list, a class roster, and CO and saliva lists. *School lists* contained every student alphabetically arranged within a particular school. These were used by data collection teams in the field on collection day to keep track of students who might have transferred to new classes. This also enabled collectors to include students who were consented to participate.

Classroom rosters were obtained from the school as close to the collection date as possible to eliminate extra work in the classroom. This information provided the exact classroom, teacher and period, for each student. It was usually after this information had been entered into the computer that ID numbers were assigned. From this information a TNT class list was generated with consent information for each class to be measured.

CO sheets were used for data collector ratings and to record the results of the CO chemical validation measure. In addition, they served as secondary class lists. The vitalograph was used to measure the amount of carbon monoxide in a student's breath. *Saliva sheets* served as secondary class lists and were used to simplify data collector ratings of IDs of those students who completed these data.

NOTES

1. This section was contributed by Sande Craig.
2. This section was contributed by Ms. Custer-Smith.

NINE

Prevention Program Evaluation

This chapter presents the implementation, process, and outcomes evaluation of the prevention trial in Project TNT. First, definitions of what are meant by each of these terms as they relate to tobacco use prevention research are provided. Subjects in these three types of evaluation are described next, followed by a description of the data analytic approaches taken, and a summary of the results obtained in the prevention project at immediate posttest, 1-year posttest (along with consideration of booster effects), and 2-year posttest.

IMPLEMENTATION, PROCESS, AND OUTCOMES IN PROGRAM EVALUATION: DEFINITIONS

In the development of curricula for the present project, considerable effort was expended to derive theoretically driven but practically feasible program components linked to the experimental conditions outlined earlier. The next step in this research program was the evaluation of the major confounding variables that might hamper the adequate evaluation of program effects. Because random assignment of schools to conditions was performed, the major potential confounds involved control of program implementation, process, and condition discriminant validity (Sussman, Dent, Stacy, Hodgson, et al., 1993; Sussman, Dent, Stacy, Sun, et al., 1993).

Implementation Evaluation

This evaluation considers whether program activities were completed as intended. One of the most likely threats to the internal validity of an experimental comparison of curricula is observed differences in implementation within and across conditions that are due not to the defining characteristics of the treatments but to extraneous or unintended differences between curricula. It is desirable, therefore, to document that treatments are implemented as intended and do not deviate measurably from the original intention. Key measures in the school-based prevention context include student attendance, homework return rate, and delivery fidelity. Attendance and homework return rates are direct measures of student completion of program activities. *Delivery fidelity* measures how closely *actual* delivery of a curriculum is to its maximum *intended* delivery. *Delivery fidelity* is defined here as consisting of four levels of departure from ideal delivery: *adherence* (whether the curriculum was delivered *at all*), *exposure* (pertaining to how much of the curriculum was delivered), *reinvention* (given that the whole curriculum was delivered, whether the curriculum was delivered as written), and how *smooth the delivery* was (i.e., whether or not there were interruptions in delivery of material; see Pentz et al., 1990). Adherence refers to the most severe level of departure in the delivery of the curriculum, and smoothness of delivery refers to the most mild level of departure.

Process Evaluation

In the present context, process evaluation looks at multiple perspectives regarding measurement of the quality of a curriculum that was delivered. Process is differentiated from implementation in that it consists of subjective ratings of curriculum quality as opposed to measurement of completion of program activities. Process measures in the present school-based prevention context include student, health educator, and regular classroom teacher-observer perceptions of class control, class enthusiasm, understandability of curriculum lessons, health educator effectiveness and enthusiasm, and perceived overall curriculum effectiveness. Ideally, process ratings are favorable and equivalent across conditions. If they are, it is likely that future behavioral effects on the students will be due to curricula content differences and not to curriculum credibility effects (Sussman, Dent, Brannon, et al., 1989).

Outcomes Evaluation

This evaluation considers the effectiveness of a program on achieving immediate and long-term goals. One main immediate goal in the present context is to assess whether a program has adequately imparted its content matter to the participants. An evaluation of knowledge items completed at immediate posttest permits an assessment of whether students have learned central concepts within a condition and whether discriminant validity of program material is achieved when comparing different conditions. The main long-term goal of a project in the present context is to assess preventive effects on tobacco use behavior. Behavioral effects among adolescents are examined at least 1 year after implementation of a program because the statistical power to detect changes in behavior usually demands this time lag or longer (Flay, 1985).

Sources of Data for the Prevention Analysis

Measures of implementation relied primarily on health educators' reports of attendance, homework received, and delivery fidelity, because health educators are best able to provide these reports. On the other hand, three sources of ratings were available for process measures: the students, the health educators, and the teacher-observers. The health educators were those persons who were hired and trained by others in Project TNT. They had no connection to the schools they visited other than to deliver the curriculum. When a health educator taught a curriculum, the regular classroom teacher observed the delivery but did not contribute to it in any way. Thus three perspectives were represented in the process evaluation. The students provided ratings from the perspective of a program recipient, the health educator provided ratings from the perspective of a delivery person, and the classroom teacher provided ratings from the perspective of an observer. Finally, the posttest knowledge evaluation, 1-year behavior outcomes, and 2-year behavior outcomes relied on students' ratings because students are the targets of the project. The contents of these measures were described in Chapter 8.

DATA

Student Immediate Posttest and Follow-Up Data

Immediate posttest data were collected the next school day after completion of a 10-day curriculum (or simply 11 days later in the control condition), from 6,716 seventh-grade students, of whom 50% were male. Regarding ethnic composition, 60% were white, 27% were Hispanic, 7% were black, and 6% were Asian or "other." One-year follow-up data were collected from 7,052 students. Ninety-three percent of the students reported attending the same school 1 year earlier. Two-year follow-up data were collected from 7,219 students. These students were now 9th graders in high school. Sixty-five percent of the students reported having attended a Project TNT junior high school the previous year. Data were aggregated to the school level at each time point, using the total school sample.

Students consisted of two cohorts. In Cohort 1, students from all 7th-grade classes at 20 schools were followed on an individual level. In Cohort 2, students from 28 other schools were followed as a repeated cross-sectional random sampling of 7th-grade classes. Posttest data, 1-year follow-up data, and 2-year follow-up data from the full sample are presented here.

When reaching 9th grade, students from all but one school (which was a kindergarten through 12th-grade school) transferred to local high schools. Follow-up becomes much more difficult when subjects switch to new schools. Several items have been used to try to follow up project subjects when data collection "sweeps" across 9th-grade classrooms. Simply asking subjects if they have completed questionnaires or were part of a prevention program over the last 2 years is a useful method, but one subject to an acquiescence effect (people tend to say "yes"). Requesting information learned in previous programming or about the name of the organization the data collection team was from (for control students) is another method; however, a gross underrepresentation of project students tends to result. The method capable of reaching over 80% of project students is one that simply asks students for the names of the schools they attended last year. Thus a one-page list of schools was included in Project TNT that requested this information. The students simply checked the school they had attended previously. Cohort 1 students were matched by their identification numbers as well as previous school attended; tracking of Cohort 2 students relied only on previous school attended.

At each wave of collection, students from the individual-level cohort had breath or saliva samples collected and were read a script that informed them that their data were confidential. Students from the grade-level cohort did not provide biochemical samples, and were read a script that informed them that the data collected were anonymous. Both of these procedures have been shown to increase the accuracy of self-reported tobacco use. Students were instructed that they were not expected to complete the full questionnaire. Rather, they were told to complete as many items that they were able to in the one class period. Students were requested to stop completing any other items 5 minutes before the end of the period and were instructed to complete the *program evaluation items*. For those from whom biochemical data were collected, these biochemical data were not analyzed because of cost (for the saliva data) and incomplete completion (completion only among 20 of 48 schools; individual-level cohort).

Health Educator Data

Implementation and process data were collected at immediate posttest from nine core project health educators, who were equally represented across conditions and each of whom had taught each curriculum at least once. Of these health educators, 78% were white, 11% were black (one educator), and 11% were Latina (one educator). All were female. All health educators received 3 weeks of training (120 hours) before delivering a curriculum. Mean age was 28 years (SD = 2.7 years).

Teacher-Observer Data

Process data were collected at immediate posttest from 76 teacher-observers, the regular classroom teachers who observed the curriculum delivery process. All teachers from those 7th-grade classes in which a curriculum was delivered completed the teacher data. Of these teachers, approximately 85% were white and 51% were female. Mean age was approximately 35 years (SD = 10 years).

ANALYSIS

Implementation, process, and posttest knowledge analyses were accomplished through use of one-way analyses of variance (ANOVAs) examining the response means from the conditions. If an ANOVA model was significant, least significant difference (LSD) post hoc comparisons were calculated between pairs of means. The LSD post hoc test controls for the comparisonwise alpha error rate at .05 for comparisons of any two means within a set of means. For example, in a comparison in which the four program conditions may differ in mean level of perceived effectiveness, the LSD comparison reveals which of the conditions show a significant difference between mean perceived effectiveness from any of the other conditions. All statistics were calculated at the school level of analysis.

Of principal interest in this study is the change in prevalence of tobacco use over the 1-year study interval (posttest to 1-year follow-up) and 2-year study interval (posttest to 2-year follow-up). We constructed four behavior outcome measures—two that measured the change in rates of initial trial of cigarettes and smokeless tobacco, and two that indicated the change in rates of weekly use of these substances (described in Chapter 8). Measures were constructed at the school level as the difference in observed school-level prevalence (follow-up minus the initial rate). The number of subjects measured at each school was then used as a weighing factor in all subsequent calculations (i.e., small schools contributed less weight). At 2-year follow-up we conducted the same type of analysis using 2-year data.

We first examined the overall prevalence of tobacco use at two time points and the change in prevalence by gender and region. At each time point, and for the difference, we calculated a least squares means t test between regions (urban versus rural) and between genders (male versus female), with school as the unit of analysis. In the case of gender comparisons, each school contributed a separate mean for the males and the females at the school. For urban versus rural comparisons, each school contributed a single mean. These analyses were used to test for different prevalence at each time point in the regions and between the two genders as well as to test for differential increase in use in these subpopulations.

We then examined the effects of the four curricula on each of our tobacco outcome measures by computing a five-group one-way analysis of covariance (ANCOVA) model with school as the unit of analysis. Two covariates were included, the blocking composite assignment variable and a measure of school "turnover" defined as the proportion of new students at the school at the 1- or 2-year follow-up (average value = 7%). These two covariates were added to the models to reduce the observed error variance between schools and increase the power of the analysis rather than as "adjustments" for group imbalances. Interaction terms between gender and treatment, and region and treatment, also were calculated; however, neither term was significant in posttest to 1-year, or posttest to 2-year, models, and they were subsequently dropped. This result indicates that any pattern of treatment effects found is (statistically) the same across gender and region. Although gender-by-treatment interactions were not found (statistically) for smokeless tobacco use measures, any effect on weekly use would be totally accounted for by the males because few females were weekly users (e.g., 15 females were weekly users in 8th grade).

By using the ANCOVA model at the school level, we have assumed that the effects of the intervention are additive in the scale of changes in school proportions (i.e., each school in a group responds the same way, on average, to each type of treatment) and that rate of change without any systematic intervention can be characterized as a constant that is estimated by the control schools. We therefore calculated planned least-square mean difference comparisons between each of the four treatment group means and the control group mean, using the ANCOVA model error term, for each behavioral outcome measure. In addition, we compared all possible pairs of group means in a post hoc fashion to determine if treatments dominated each other.

IMPLEMENTATION RESULTS

Adherence did not vary by condition, and the curricula were implemented at all schools. *Exposure* to the curricula did not vary by condition; all activities were completed in each curriculum. Results for the remainder of the implementation items are summarized as follows (also see Sussman, Dent, Stacy, Hodgson, et al., 1993). Reported by the health educators, the least *reinvention* was in the informational social influence condition, whereas the other three program conditions did not differ. The most *smooth delivery* was in the physical consequences condition, the least smooth delivery was in the combined condition, and the other two conditions did not differ. Student attendance, as indicated on attendance records, averaged approximately 90% across conditions, equivalent to the average attendance in the regular classroom situation, and attendance was slightly but significantly higher in the physical consequences condition compared to the informational and normative social influences conditions, which did not differ (but not the combined condition).

Health educators reported that the highest homework return rates were in the combined and physical consequences conditions, and the lowest return rates were in the informational and normative social influences conditions. Students' report of homework return averaged about 85%, and was 10% higher than actual homework return as recorded by the health educator. Like the health educators, students reported relatively higher homework return rates in the combined and physical consequences conditions.

PROCESS RESULTS

Students

On an average index of 21 adjectives describing the program, the physical consequences condition was rated most favorably, although all treatment conditions were rated moderately favorably and the physical consequences condition was not rated significantly higher than the informational social influence condition. Class enthusiasm was rated lowest by students in the normative social influence condition, although only significantly lower than the physical consequences and combined conditions. Perceived program effectiveness, recommendation of program to others, and perceived program usefulness were rated by students in the physical consequences condition as significantly higher than in the other three conditions, which did not differ.

Health Educators

Contrary to the students, health educators rated all conditions more equally. Class control, understandability, and perceived effectiveness did not differ by experimental condition. Health educator enthusiasm and effort, and class enthusiasm, did differ by condition. Health educators reported the least enthusiasm for teaching the normative social influences condition as compared to the combined and physical consequences conditions. Health educators' judgments of students enthusiasm were highest in the physical consequences condition. Health educator judgments of teaching effort were highest in the combined condition, as compared to the other three conditions, which did not differ.

Seven of the health educators provided a ranking of overall quality of the curricula at the end of the year on the curriculum evaluation form. On this ranking the combined condition was rated most favorably, although agreement of the rankings among health educators was fairly low (Kendall's $W = .27$).

Teacher-Observers

Likewise, the classroom teachers did not differ across conditions in their ratings of class control or understandability. On the other hand, they also did *not* differ in their ratings across conditions of class and teacher enthusiasm. Teacher-observers in the physical consequences condition did show a significantly higher rating of perceived effectiveness than those in the normative social influence condition, although the remaining two program conditions did not differ from either the physical consequences or normative social influence conditions.

KNOWLEDGE OUTCOMES

Although the posttest percentage correct on the knowledge items averaged around 50%, the relative difference between groups was significantly different—in line with the content of the items. For example, the highest score on the normative social influence knowledge items was attained by those students in the normative social influence condition (67% correct). Program conditions that were not provided normative social influence information obtained knowledge scores that did not differ from the control condition (51%-54% correct). Also, scores in the combined condition were in between those for each single-component condition (59% correct). This latter result is expected because students in that condition received less material, but from all curricula. Thus, as intended, the different conditions manipulated different domains of knowledge, indicating content discriminant validity of the conditions.

BEHAVIOR OUTCOMES AT 1 YEAR POSTPROGRAM

Within-Time Prevalence by Gender and Region

Immediate posttest and 1-year follow-up for cigarette use did not differ by gender, although trial and weekly use of smokeless tobacco use did differ. Use of smokeless tobacco was higher among males. Regarding region, trial of cigarette smoking and smokeless tobacco use was higher in the rural schools than in the urban schools at both time points. Regular use of tobacco products did not differ by region.

Change in Prevalence by Gender and Region

From immediate posttest to the 1-year follow-up, trial and weekly use prevalence of cigarettes rose about 8% and 3%, respectively, an equal percentage among males and females. On the other hand, trial and weekly use prevalence of smokeless tobacco rose only for males (5% change for trial use and 1% change for weekly use).

Cigarette use prevalence rose equally across urban and rural regions (about 8% and 3% change for trial and regular use, respectively). Trial of smokeless tobacco rose about 3% at urban schools and about 1% at rural schools, whereas weekly use increased only about 0.5% at both regions, which did not differ from each other (see Table 9.1).

Change in Prevalence by Condition

Change in prevalence data comparing the program and control conditions from immediate posttest to the 1-year follow-up are shown in Table 9.2. For both trial and weekly use of cigarettes, the informational social influence, physical consequences, and combined conditions (which did not differ from each other) were superior to the normative social influence and control conditions

Table 9.1 Prevalence of Tobacco Use Over Time: By Gender and
Region (Grades 7 to 8)

	Trial Use			Weekly Use		
	Immediate Posttest	1-Year Follow-Up	Difference	Immediate Posttest	1-Year Follow-Up	Difference
Cigarettes						
Total	.40	.47	.080	.06	.09	.033
Male	$.41^a$	$.48^a$	$.071^a$	$.06^a$	$.09^a$	$.030^a$
Female	$.38^a$	$.47^a$	$.093^a$	$.06^a$	$.10^a$	$.036^a$
Urban	$.35^a$	$.44^a$	$.090^a$	$.05^a$	$.08^a$	$.032^a$
Rural	$.43^b$	$.50^b$	$.071^a$	$.07^a$	$.11^a$	$.034^a$
Smokeless Tobacco						
Total	.08	.10	.020	.01	.01	.004
Male	$.12^a$	$.17^a$	$.054^a$	$.02^a$	$.03^a$	$.008^a$
Female	$.04^b$	$.04^b$	$.002^b$	$.00^b$	$.00^b$	$.000^b$
Urban	$.05^a$	$.08^a$	$.029^a$	$.01^a$	$.01^a$	$.004^a$
Rural	$.10^b$	$.11^b$	$.010^b$	$.01^a$	$.02^a$	$.005^a$

NOTE: Within each column (within gender or region comparisons), significant differences ($p <$ .05, two-tailed) between percentages are indicated by different-letter superscripts; same-letter superscripts denote no significant difference.

(which did not differ from each other). For trial of smokeless tobacco use, the normative social influence, physical consequences, and combined conditions (which did not differ from each other) were superior to the informational social influence and control conditions (which did not differ from each other). For weekly use of smokeless tobacco, the combined condition was superior to all other conditions (which did not differ from each other).

BOOSTER EFFECTS

The issue of program effects "fading" over time was addressed in Project TNT by delivering a program booster and evaluating its short-term effectiveness. Immediately following the 1-year follow-up survey, students in the four active treatment conditions were presented with 2 days of "booster" lessons. The lessons reviewed material specific to the curriculum received in the previous year.

Table 9.2　Treatment Effects From Project TNT: Change in Prevalence of Tobacco Use (Grades 7 to 8)

	Condition				
		Informational Normative			Standard
		Social	Social	Physical	Care
Tobacco Measure	Combined	Influence	Influence	Consequences	Control
Trial cigarette use	.073[b]	.071[b]	.102[a]	.061[b]	.093[a]
Weekly cigarette use	.020[b]	.032[b]	.053[a]	.026[b]	.056[a]
Trial smokeless tobacco use	.017[b]	.035[a]	.026[b]	.024[b]	.041[a]
Weekly smokeless tobacco use	−.004[b]	.005[a]	.003[a]	.006[a]	.005[a]

SOURCE: "Project Towards No Tobacco Use: One-Year Behavior Outcomes" by S. Sussman, C. W. Dent, A. W. Stacy, P. Sun, S. Craig, T. R. Simon, D. Burton, and B. R. Flay, 1993, *American Journal of Public Health, 83*, pp. 1245-1250. Copyright © 1993 by the American Public Health Association. Adapted by permission.

NOTE: Within each row comparison, significant differences (p < .05, two-tailed) between percentages are indicated by different-letter superscripts; same-letter superscripts denote no significant difference.

The use of booster lessons to supplement a classroom prevention program also may significantly enhance program effects, especially when repeated over a number of years (Flay et al., 1989), and has been a feature in advanced-generation primary prevention studies (e.g., Flay, 1985; also see Chapter 7). Messages that are repeated over relatively long periods of time, and that allow expression of newly formed attitudes and behaviors, are relatively likely to be incorporated into one's personal repertoire (Flay, 1981; Flay et al., 1983); thus a reasonably inclusive booster period for each curriculum seems appropriate (Botvin et al., 1983; Flay et al., 1985). Booster lessons (a) summarize previously taught material, (b) review and practice key components of previous programming (e.g., role playing, decision making, making a public commitment not to use tobacco), and (c) encourage discussion of how program material was used in postprogram daily living (Flay et al., 1989; Silvestri & Flay, 1989). Classroom discussion, small group work, and role-play exercises are the methods used to exchange information. Generally, little new information is provided in a one- or two-lesson booster program.

In Project TNT, booster programming was provided 1 year postprogram (8th grade). Four separate curricula were developed, one for each study condition. The four booster curricula each contain similar process elements in the first and second lessons. The activities in Lessons 1 and 2 take the same amount of time, use a "Jeopardy" game, involve recall of experiences from the last year, and involve skills practice or situation enhancement via role plays. The content of the lessons of each curriculum address either (a) normative social influence, (b) informational social influence, (c) physical consequences, or (d) combined normative and informational social influences plus physical consequences.

In Lesson 1 of all four curricula, the students are divided into teams and play a game very similar to that of the television game show "Jeopardy." Students are asked questions specific to the curriculum they received last year. Students also are provided with written information about the 10 lessons they had received previously.

In Lesson 2, the following activities are reviewed and practiced. In the normative social influence curriculum, students review the various aspects of peer pressure and assertively saying "no" to drug offers, learn to handle stressful peer pressure situations by being prepared, and practice these skills through role playing. In the informational social influence curriculum, students recall material including building up self-esteem, learning social-situation-oriented decision-making skills, understanding and combating advertisements and other media influences, and communicating more effectively. These skills are practiced through role playing. In the physical consequences curriculum, students discuss the physical consequences of tobacco use, and students role-play situations involving the various diseases and problems associated with tobacco use, such as wasting money, addiction, harming others, and getting lung cancer. Finally, in the combined condition, students focus on the multiple aspects of the previous year's instruction. Activities elicit information from the students that helps them to recall what they had learned about refusing tobacco offers, communicating more effectively, building self-esteem, combating media influences and advertisements, and becoming more personally aware of physical consequences from tobacco use. Again, skills are practiced through role playing.

A postbooster survey was collected on approximately 1,500 students. The survey contained drug use intention items (tobacco, alcohol, marijuana), curriculum content knowledge items, and ratings of classroom management and program usefulness. Two sets of analyses were performed. In Set 1 we examined the need for program boosting by comparing 1-year follow-up (prebooster) responses across conditions. Analysis consisted of comparing means of each of the four treatment conditions to the control condition using ANCOVA with area (urban/rural), sex, and the blocking assignment variable as covariates. In Set 2 we examined booster effects by comparing pre- to postbooster change across conditions. The later was accomplished with ANCOVA models that included matched prebooster items as covariates.

Results from Set 1 analyses indicated that except in a few instances, knowledge gains seen at immediate postprogram had decayed on items from each of three content areas (12 items total, 4 per each content area). The program conditions differed from the standard care control condition only in that more boys recalled that smokeless tobacco is as addictive as cigarettes from lessons in the physical consequences and combined conditions than from lessons in the other conditions, and more girls recalled the name of a young athlete who died from oral cancer from those same lessons than from lessons in the other conditions. More girls in the combined condition also understood the definition of "reverse the pressure" than girls in the control condition. Intentions to use drugs were also fairly comparable across program and control conditions at 1 year, indicating a fading of program effects on attitudes. The exceptions were that girls from the combined curriculum had lower intention to use cigarettes than control girls, and both boys and girls who received the combined curriculum indicated that they had a lower intention to use marijuana than controls. These results are not necessarily inconsistent with 1-year behavioral effects because intentions measure a different construct than current behavior. In this case intentions to use in the distant future were being measured, with averages varying between "some time after high school" to "never" response categories.

Set 2 analyses, which assessed the effectiveness of the booster, revealed an interesting pattern of results. First, we found that rating of program helpfulness and rating of classroom management did not differ between program conditions. This allowed us to interpret the results without process or expectancy confounds (Sussman, Dent, Stacy, Hodgson, et al., 1993). Regarding knowledge gains, students generally exhibited gains in the areas to which they had been exposed. For example, students from the normative social influence condition showed gains on normative social influence knowledge items but not on physical consequence or informational social influence knowledge items. Students in the combined condition gained in all three areas. As for behavioral intentions, the booster effects were limited to those in the informational social influence condition regarding smoking of cigarettes, girls in the informational social influence condition regarding smokeless tobacco use, students in the combined curriculum condition regarding alcohol use (not explicitly mentioned in the booster), and boys in the normative social influence condition regarding marijuana use (marijuana was not addressed in the curriculum). In summary, it would appear that booster lessons do need to be applied because knowledge and long-term behavioral intention gains appear to fade after a 1-year interval. The actual behavior effects of the booster need to be tested with longer follow-up data.

BEHAVIOR OUTCOMES AT 2 YEARS POSTPROGRAM

Within-Time Prevalence and Change in Prevalence
by Gender and Region

Change in prevalence of tobacco use data for trial of cigarettes between 8th and 9th grades was 9% overall. Change did not vary by gender or region. More triers of cigarettes were in rural than urban regions, 60% versus 52% in 9th grade. Change in trial of smokeless tobacco use was small (2% overall), which did not vary by gender or region. More males than females were triers of smokeless tobacco, 20% versus 4% in 9th grade, and more triers were in rural than urban regions, 12% versus 9% in 9th grade. Change in weekly cigarette smoking was 5% overall, which did

Table 9.3 More Treatment Effects From Project TNT: Change in Prevalence of Tobacco Use (Grades 7 to 9)

	Condition				
		Informational Normative			Standard
		Social	Social	Physical	Care
Tobacco Measure	Combined	Influence	Influence	Consequences	Control
Trial cigarette use	.16[b]	.15[b]	.17[b]	.13[b]	.23[a]
Weekly cigarette use	.04[b]	.12[a]	.09[a]	.08[a]	.09[a]
Trial smokeless tobacco use	.07[a]	.04[a]	.04[a]	.00[b]	.07[a]
Weekly smokeless tobacco use	−.00[ab]	.02[a]	.02[a]	−.01[b]	.01[a]

SOURCE: Dent et al., 1994.
NOTE: Within each row comparison, significant differences (p < .05, two-tailed) between percentages are indicated by different-letter superscripts; same-letter superscripts denote no significant difference; use of two letters indicates a marginal effect.

not vary significantly by gender or region. Weekly smoking was 14% at 9th grade, which did not vary in prevalence by gender or region. Finally, weekly smokeless tobacco use changed only slightly over 1% overall, more among males than females (7% of males but still under 1% of females were weekly users at 9th grade). Weekly smokeless tobacco use did not change by urban versus rural region. Four percent reported weekly use of smokeless tobacco in both regions at 9th grade.

Change in Prevalence by Condition

Analyses of treatment effects regarding the Year 2 follow-up data indicate support for 2-year maintenance of effects in the combined and physical consequences conditions. Boostering the program may have been of importance for maintenance of effects. These 2-year follow-up data are shown in Table 9.3, and show change in prevalence by condition from 7th to 9th grades. Over the 2-year period, all program conditions (which did not differ from each other) were superior to the standard care control condition regarding trial of cigarettes; the combined condition was superior to all other conditions (which did not differ from each other) regarding weekly smoking; the physical consequences condition was superior to all other conditions (which did not differ from each other) regarding trial use of smokeless tobacco; and the combined and physical consequences conditions were superior to the other conditions regarding weekly smokeless tobacco use. The combined condition did not differ from the physical consequences condition and did not differ *significantly* from the other conditions (also see Dent et al., 1994). Project TWT is one of three recent school-based prevention programs that show an effect on smokeless tobacco use (see U.S. DHHS, 1994 and Appendix H).

PART FOUR

Cessation Component of Project Towards No Tobacco Use (TNT)

Part Four presents the cessation component of Project TNT. Chapter 10 provides the history and theoretical basis of tobacco use cessation research, and presents the process used to develop the cessation curriculum. Chapter 11 presents the cessation clinic evaluation. Without a doubt, the discussion of cessation is much more brief than that of prevention. This is because adolescent prevention research has had a much longer research history than has adolescent cessation research. In spite of its relatively short research history, available data on cessation research are presented here in hopes that this information may stimulate further research in this area.

TEN

History, Theoretical Basis, and Program Development of Adolescent Tobacco Use Cessation Research

This chapter presents the history and theoretical basis of adolescent tobacco use cessation programming, as well as the process for cessation program development. The first section discusses available data regarding self-initiated and program-initiated cessation rates for adolescent smokeless tobacco use and cigarette smoking, and also discusses four general functions tobacco use serves for regular adolescent tobacco users. The latter information serves as a basis for the construction of the psychosocial dependency and addiction clinics that were the two program conditions in the Project TNT cessation study.

The next two sections of this chapter discuss development of the cessation recruitment and clinic content aspects of the Project TNT cessation study. A 20-page questionnaire was administered to 12 high schools in California and 12 high schools in Illinois (one class of 9th, 10th, 11th, and 12th graders, $n = 120$ students per school in California and two classes per grade, $n = 240$ students per school in Illinois) to allow a *multiyear assessment of high school grade cohorts.* This anonymous assessment was performed in Years 2, 4, and 5 of the project. This questionnaire contained many of the same items that were used in the prevention questionnaire, including grade-level tobacco use information. In addition, items such as stages of readiness to quit and reasons for quitting tobacco use were included in this questionnaire. This large-scale assessment thus provided one source of clinic development information as well as a behavior context for evaluating school-based clinic cessation rates.

Cessation development also involved *small-scale assessments* in Year 1, *recruitment development* in Year 2, *cessation clinic content development* in Year 3, and *cessation intervention* implementation and 3-month follow-up in Year 4. Year 1 assessment study results are discussed in detail in Chapters 4 and 6 of this book as part of the prevention study development. Within the context of cessation, one may summarize the results of the assessment studies by mentioning that regular tobacco use is concentrated in certain groups (high-risk youth), although tobacco is used regularly throughout the student body (Project TNT Group Names Study). Both physiological and social effects might need to be considered for counteraction in cessation efforts (Project TNT school personnel and student interviews), and it is feasible the cessation clinics should address both the use of smokeless tobacco and the use of cigarettes (Project TNT school personnel and student interviews, and Group Names Study).

The size and number of pilot tests in Illinois were equivalent to those in California. The large-scale questionnaire sample size, however, was twice as large in Illinois because our programmatic efforts there were fairly recent, and we had few alternative sources to establish reliability of tobacco use estimates at that time. One other main difference in sampling is that three schools were selected from very rural farming communities in southern Illinois. Anecdotal reports of very high rates of smokeless tobacco use led to our acquisition of these schools as a convenient sample. The results obtained in pilot studies and in the main trial were nearly identical across sites. Although cessation results do not vary, attention paid to smokeless tobacco use versus cigarette smoking in the pilot tests and clinics was greater in the three southern Illinois schools.

HISTORY AND THEORETICAL BASIS

History

Recent programs based on social psychological processes, as described above, have been moderately successful at reducing onset of smokeless tobacco use (Elder et al., 1993; Severson et al., 1991; Sussman, Dent, Stacy, Sun, et al., 1993; see Appendix H) and cigarette smoking (Flay, 1985; Flay et al., 1983; Perry et al., 1983; Perry, Killen, Telch, Stinkard, & Danaher, 1980). However, there are almost no data describing cessation processes or evaluating cessation interventions for adolescents who already are either regular smokeless tobacco users or regular cigarette smokers (U.S. DHHS, 1994; also see Appendix H summary of adolescent cessation programs). In fact, for smokeless tobacco, there are virtually no data for cessation programs even for adult users. One early report (Glover, 1986) on two pilot smokeless tobacco cessation clinics for 18- to 22-year-olds modeled after a smoking cessation program found only a 2.3% 6-month point-prevalence quit rate for smokeless tobacco, compared to earlier findings of up to a 38% quit rate for cigarette cessation clinics. These data suggested a dismal prospect for future smokeless tobacco cessation efforts. However, the subjects in that study apparently were mandated by their university to attend the clinics and were not strongly motivated to quit. A more recent survey of 191 current male adolescent smokeless tobacco users indicated that 37% of them made self-initiated attempts to quit smokeless tobacco use but failed (Ary, Lichtenstein, Severson, Weissman, & Seeley, 1989). However, this survey was of users and did not reflect the proportion of total users who tried to quit on their own and either succeeded or did not succeed in quitting. A large-scale assessment of this sort was accomplished in Project TNT, as presented in Chapter 11.

Very few recent smokeless tobacco cessation programs with adolescents or adults have been conducted. One three-session smokeless tobacco cessation clinic program with 25 adolescents indicated a 16% point-prevalence cessation rate at 3 months postclinic (Eakin et al., 1989). One eight-session smokeless tobacco cessation clinic program with eight young male adults indicated a very high cessation rate at 9 months postclinic (six of eight participants, 75%). This study unfortunately involved no biochemical validation and a small sample, although corroborative reports were obtained (DiLorenzo, Kern, & Pieper, 1991). Another study of 42 young adults who participated in nine clinic sessions over a 5-week period resulted in a 62% overall smokeless tobacco cessation rate at 1 month postclinic, which decreased to 48% at 3 months postclinic and to 29% at 6 months postclinic (Zavela, Harrison, & Owens, 1991). Finally, minimal intervention in smokeless tobacco cessation among 576 male adults who received an oral exam, explanation of smokeless tobacco health risks, advice to stop and brief counseling, a video, and self-help material from a dentist health care provider resulted in a 10% cessation rate at a 12-month follow-up (Stevens, Severson, Lichtenstein, Little, & Leben, 1992). Other smokeless tobacco cessation projects among adults are ongoing (e.g., Margaret Walsh with college baseball and football players; Steve Sussman, Clyde Dent, and Herbert Severson with lumber mill employees). Generally, these data suggest that it may be much more difficult to stop using smokeless tobacco than to stop smoking. In sum, though, there is nothing we can say with confidence about the nature of smokeless tobacco dependency or smokeless tobacco cessation.

For cigarette smoking, three areas of research may have some relevance: (a) the few reports that exist on self-initiated or school-clinic-based adolescent smoking cessation, (b) findings from the youth prevention literature that may bear also on cessation, and (c) the literature on adult cessation. From the first area of research it has been reported that spontaneous smoking cessation attempts among high school students or young adults are not an uncommon occurrence (Hansen, Collins, Johnson, & Graham, 1985; Pallonen et al., 1990; U.S. DHHS, 1994, p. 78). As a typical example, in one survey of high school students in two California school districts, 72% of the teenage smokers reported they had recently attempted to quit smoking (Hansen, Collins, Johnson, & Graham, 1985). This figure is consistent with surveys of adults, in which approximately 80% of smokers report that they want to stop smoking (U.S. DHHS, 1984). On the other hand, another quite recent study found that as few as one out of six adolescent smokers is really ready to take action and try to quit "in the near future"

(Pallonen, Rossi, Smith, Prochaska, & Almeida, 1993). National data indicate that only between 1% and 2% of heavy lifetime adolescent smokers (> 100 cigarettes) report quitting for at least a 30-day period (U.S. DHHS, 1994, p. 69). A much higher percentage of adult smokers want to quit as soon as possible, although self-initiated cessation among adults (in California) is only 4% per year (Burns & Pierce, 1992).

Skinner et al. (1985), on the basis of an examination of 3-year panel data collected from 7th- to 12th-grade students, suggested that smoking is partly a result of the weakening of bonds to school and parents, and that for adolescents who stop smoking the break is temporary, whereas for continuing smokers the weakening continues. Peer smoking is a main predictor of continued smoking (Ary & Biglan, 1988). This fact has been taken into account in current adolescent smoking cessation programs. For example, one study compared a cognitive-behavioral group smoking cessation intervention focusing on developing students' belief in their *own* decision-making power (which presumably would counteract informational social influence effects, such as peer smoking), and found that the intervention yielded significantly greater smoking reduction than an information placebo condition (78% versus 46%, not controlling for others who increased their levels of smoking; Lotecka & MacWhinney, 1983). Likewise a study of a 2-year intensive intervention for smoking and nutrition with 13- to 15-year-old students in East Finland, which included some peer pressure resistance elements, yielded a cessation rate of 37% for boys and 35% for girls, compared to a spontaneous cessation rate of 0% for the no-treatment group (Pallonen, 1987).

Second, the literature on programs aimed at preventing the onset of smoking among youth includes occasional reports on the effects of these programs on students already smoking. For example, one study comparing a four-session social influences approach with traditional health education as a control group reported significant program effects at one year among relatively heavy daily smokers (over 10 cigarettes a day; Biglan et al., 1987). Likewise, the Project TNT prevention study demonstrated a decrease in prevalence of weekly smoking (Sussman, Dent, Stacy, Sun, et al., 1993; Chapter 9 of this book).

Third, the main difficulty in interpreting any of the few reports on smoking cessation among adolescents is in determining what "stages" of smoking behavior apply. Teenage smokers can be thought of as being in the final stages of acquisition, in which case a "youth prevention model" could apply (Flay et al., 1983), and cessation interventions could be developed based on such a model. Alternatively, once they become regular, daily smokers, adolescents could be considered to have habits comparable to those of adults, in which case an "adult cessation model" would best apply (Billings & Moos, 1983; Lichtenstein, 1982; Prochaska & DiClemente, 1983). There is a much larger research history regarding adult smoking cessation (Lichtenstein & Glasgow, 1992). Even among adults, though, the effectiveness of promising cessation approaches, such as teaching relapse prevention skills, remains in debate, and much research continues in that arena.

In summary, self-initiated cessation among adolescents is lower than among adults, but the topography of smoking in adolescence is much more dynamic (Pallonen et al., 1990). Also, there have been a few small-scale cessation programs completed with adolescents in the past with limited evaluation, and success is equal to about half that of adult programs (i.e., immediate cessation is about 20%-25%; see U.S. DHHS, 1994); almost no cessation attempts have been measured regarding smokeless tobacco use. Available studies indicate a very wide range of immediate smokeless tobacco cessation (2%-75%). One caveat when making any inferences on the basis of these smokeless tobacco studies should be mentioned; these few available studies mix results of adolescents with those of young adults. Generally, the studies on adolescents reveal relatively lower success rates. The largest smoking and smokeless tobacco cessation trial with adolescents is Project TNT, which is discussed in this chapter and in Chapter 11.

Theoretical Basis

There may be a differential importance of addiction processes versus psychosocial factors in adolescent cessation. It is unclear when youth begin to feel addicted, feel physical consequences, and desire to quit. Relevant variables probably involve daily use and withdrawal symptoms. Anywhere between 25% and 50% of older teenage tobacco users report withdrawal symptoms when attempting to quit (U.S. DHHS, 1994; Sussman, Dent, Stacy, Burton, & Flay, 1989). Teenage tobacco users are in between the younger adolescent experimenters and adult users regarding behavioral investment in tobacco use. Anecdotal evidence prior to the Project TNT cessation trial suggests that smokeless tobacco use may be more difficult to stop than cigarette smoking (Glover, 1986); other evidence, however, suggests that differences in chemical addiction properties for regular use of smokeless tobacco versus cigarettes might not be significant (Gritz et al., 1981). Clearly, smokeless tobacco use is *at least as* addicting as cigarette smoking (U.S. DHHS, 1989). There are at least four theoretical models that could provide a basis for an adolescent cessation intervention. Burton, Sussman, Dent, et al. (1989) and Burton (1994) place these four models in a hypothesized sequence of tobacco use acquisition. First, social influences predominate as reasons for using tobacco. Next, addiction to nicotine becomes a main reason for use. Third, psychosocial dependency becomes of major importance. Finally, negative affect becomes a main reason to use tobacco. Adolescent cessation of tobacco use is likely to be most successful when considering the factors most potent to adolescents. All four reasons for tobacco use, but particularly the latter factors, operate for adults. Perhaps, for adolescents, on the other hand, earlier factors predominate. Content of cessation programming to counteract these four factors is summarized briefly as follows.

1. *The social influences model,* as described above for the prevention component of this study (e.g., Sussman, 1989), incorporates both normative and informational social influence elements. It has as its key concepts (a) the development of skills to resist a variety of social approval factors presumed to obstruct the cessation process, and (b) the identification of strategies for developing expressions of group values and belongingness as alternatives to tobacco use.

2. *The chemical addiction model* (Leventhal & Cleary, 1980; Pollin, 1985; Russell, 1986) has as its key concept the breaking of an addiction, including going through a withdrawal period with cravings, physical symptoms, and so on. Chemical addiction is sometimes thought

of as a key component in the final stages of youth acquisition of smoking (Flay et al., 1983); if this is the case, then an intervention based on a chemical addiction model could be particularly effective with teenagers who have just recently become regular tobacco users. This model might be particularly effective in cessation of smokeless tobacco (Glover, 1986).

3. *The psychosocial dependency model* (Benfari, Ecker, Ockene, & McIntyre, 1982; Burton, 1978; Green, 1977; Pechacek & Danaher, 1979) has as its key concept the identification of strategies for replacing the personal and individualized meanings of tobacco use for an individual with constructive ego-enhancing alternatives. This model primarily deals with expectations of negative consequences of cessation (e.g., failure, tension, loneliness, inability to cope). Furthermore, this model strongly indicates the role that duration of smoking plays in increasing the functional complexity, and presumably the intensity, of the dependency.

4. *The negative affect model* (Tomkins, 1966): although some researchers might place this model sequentially as operating to maintain tobacco use behavior prior to addiction, we theorized it as a final stage. In our version of this model, people use tobacco to cope with stress or feelings of upset. For a while, tobacco works to decrease negative affect. Then it stops working. Decreasing functionality of tobacco use may cause even more upset. Emotional upset is a major reason for cessation attempts among heavy smokers (Linn & Stein, 1985) and for relapse to smoking (Shiffman, 1986). It is at this stage that continuing to smoke is uncomfortable, yet stopping is quite difficult. Alternative means of coping with negative affect, such as seeking social support, reinterpretation of negative feelings as natural, and positive-affect-inducing alternatives (e.g., meditation, relaxation, exercise) are recommended.

The social influences model overlaps in part with the psychosocial dependency and negative affect models in that to avoid loneliness or to cope with negative feelings, a youth may yield to peer group pressure and use tobacco. Also, psychosocial dependency and coping with negative affect through smoking are likely to be learned initially through social informational sources. Still, these latter two models are distinct because psychosocial dependency and negative affect coping deal more with internalized, now intrapsychic, functions of tobacco use (e.g., smoking by oneself and feeling less lonely), whereas social influence theories deal more with sociological, social psychological, and noninternalized or becoming-internalized functions.

PROJECT TNT DEVELOPMENTAL STUDIES OF TOBACCO CESSATION RECRUITMENT AND SUGGESTIONS FOR CLINIC CONTENTS

Cessation motivational recruitment went through three main phases of development. First, material was used from Year 2 focus groups and large-scale questionnaire data to tap basic recruitment and other cessation-related issues. Second, a recruitment development study was accomplished. Finally, pilot testing of curricula was accomplished, which also varied use of different recruitment strategies. The structure and results of the recruitment (and clinic) development studies were nearly identical across sites. To ease presentation, mostly data from California are presented.

Focus Groups (Round 1)—The California Sample

Three high schools were assessed, one rural and two urban. One class from each grade at each school was broken down into two groups, resulting in a total of 24 possible focus groups (8 to 15 students per group). Audiotape record data were collected regarding conversations about two questions, motivating students to join a cessation group and motivating students to quit smoking or smokeless tobacco use. Four of the tapes were inaudible at a coding stage, and thus a total of 20 focus groups were coded. A finite number of responses were obtained for each of these two questions. Of the 17 motivational reasons for *joining* reported across focus groups, responses mentioned by at least half of the groups were taken as popular responses (i.e., 10 of 20 groups generated a given reason). These included keeping clinics private ($n = 12$ groups), involving social support systems ($n = 12$), making clinics a social/recreational event ($n = 11$), bringing in outside speakers ($n = 11$), and making clinics that are novel/not just talk ($n = 10$). Motivational reasons for quitting, popular and near-popular responses, included disease knowledge ($n = 20$), peer pressure to quit ($n = 14$), difficulties dating ($n = 12$), short-term physical consequences ($n = 11$), cost ($n = 9$), and addiction ($n = 7$). In general, responses were consistent over grades and regions (urban versus rural). Again, a similar sample, procedure, and results were obtained in Illinois.

Focus Groups (Round 2)

Focus groups used the material collected in the first round and developed more specific questions for probing in subsequent groups. In all cases, questioning consisted of open-ended questions to minimize facilitator bias. In Round 2, a series of 21 questions were asked of students. These questions were placed in two "sets." Set 1 emphasizes social-support-related variables pertaining to cessation, whereas Set 2 emphasizes varying incentives for making attempts to quit. These two sets are as follows.

Set 1

1. Several students have suggested that coming to a quit clinic would be embarrassing. What is embarrassing about it?
   a. People knowing you use tobacco?
   b. People knowing you want to quit?
   c. The idea that you join a group?
   d. How can we make it less embarrassing?
2. If you were a tobacco user, would you prefer a self-help program, or coming to a group?
3. If a tobacco user had access to an audiocassette self-help tape, do you think that would work? Would the person listen to the tape?
4. If the clinic were a group format, would you prefer to concentrate on yourself, or to work together as a team?
   a. Would you like a group that emphasized caring about one another and helping, or would you prefer to work alone?
   b. If a caring group is preferred, how can we encourage caring about the other group members?
5. What do you think about the idea of having a physical assessment during the first meeting (running scores, CO test) that the whole group gets a score for; then everyone would work together to make the group score better?
6. Some students have suggested that a group should have a high level of trust. How can a group develop trust? Would that be important to you?

7. Several students have suggested that people who come to the quit clinic should have buddies or helpers. How would that work?
   a. Should the buddies be users?
   b. Should they be nonusers?
   c. What about users who are not trying to quit?
   d. Does everyone have to have a buddy? or
   e. How would they get the buddy? Friend or assigned?
8. Is someone who already uses tobacco likely to encourage or discourage someone who is trying to quit?
9. Some students have suggested having ex-tobacco-users as speakers. How would that work?
   a. How old?
   b. What would the benefit be to the group?
   c. Is it necessary? or
   d. Should they lead the group or just come in once?

Set 2

1. If you were a tobacco user, would you prefer a quit clinic after school, or during the school hours? Why?
2. What do you think about the idea of a quit competition between schools?
3. Some students have suggested that quitters receive class credit for quitting. Does that present a problem with confidentiality? Is it okay if the teachers know who quit?
4. Some people have suggested that there be a party for those who quit. How would that work?
   a. Would the party be at the beginning of the clinic?
   b. Would it be a reward at the end?
   c. If it was at the end, would you tell everyone ahead of time?
5. Some students have suggested that they would quit using tobacco for sports or because of jobs they may have in the future. What do you think about the idea of having a quit clinic right before a particular sports season, say football? What about quit clinics as part of preparation for enhancing job performance?
6. What do you think about the idea of having a doctor in the quit clinic?
7. Some people have said that they quit because they know someone with a tobacco-related disease. What would motivate someone to quit who did not know someone with a tobacco-related disease? Would seeing a film with people with emphysema affect you?

8. What are the health problems that would motivate a young person to quit?

9. Does the idea that you probably will not be able to use tobacco in the workplace when you get a job matter to you?

10. Imagine that you were a tobacco user who just quit. What would you spend the money on?

11. What do you think about the idea of putting up posters in the bathrooms?

    a. Would anyone see the posters in the bathrooms?

    b. What do you think?

    c. Would they be ripped down?

    d. What would people say about them?

12. Some students have said they use tobacco because they are bored. Can you tell me more about that?

In California, four focus groups were run, one per grade at one rural high school. Four focus groups were run in Illinois as well, one per grade at one rural high school. Students gave consistent responses across sites. These data were consistent with the Round 1 data, and provided more specifics regarding issues to consider when attempting to motivate youths to join cessation clinics. Some youth reported that they would feel embarrassed to come to a clinic if they thought friends would see them and it would strain their relationship (which might center on tobacco use), and if it indicated that they were admitting they needed help. Use of confidential class release forms would help them maintain confidentiality to attend a clinic. Youth wanted to meet in groups, did not like the idea of self-help audiotapes, liked the idea of buddy systems, disliked the use of health screening as a means of assessment or as a device to encourage involvement in a clinic, disliked involvement of tobacco users who did not intend to quit, thought clinics should be held during school hours, thought there should not be a quit competition between schools, approved of receiving class credit for attending a clinic if cheating could be controlled for (i.e., nonusers who become or say they are users to get the class credit), and disliked having the clinic serve a recreational purpose (party). Also, they were not enthusiastic about having a doctor participate as a speaker or advisor in the clinics, but were enthu-

siastic about seeing a young person with a tobacco-related consequence serve as a speaker or to be shown a videotape of such a
person. To provide notice for a forthcoming clinic, students reported that posters should be put up in classrooms, not the washrooms (where they'd be ripped down). Many different types of
tobacco use consequences and monetary alternatives to purchasing tobacco were mentioned as being worthwhile topics to bring
up in clinics.

Focus Groups (Rounds 1 and 2)—
Project TNT Focus Group Effects Study

Recently, applied social researchers have shown an increased
interest in use of focus groups as a method of generating ideas and
solutions pertaining to various social problems. Yet caution in use
of this methodology is warranted because focus groups may
induce certain group effects that may bias responses.

Project TNT took the opportunity to study the operation of
group effects in focus groups because it used a focus group method
of generating clinic ideas. One major collective norm effect is the
group polarization effect. The very fact of being involved in a group
may bias subjects to respond in more extreme ways (Eiser, 1980;
Runkel & McGrath, 1972, pp. 224-226). For example, the novelty
of focus group discussion may lead participants to be more favorably disposed to stated hypotheses or solutions to social problems
after material is discussed in the group than when it is generated
on a pregroup questionnaire.

On the other hand, one of the stated advantages of focus groups is
that of producing a synergistic group effect (Stewart & Shamdasani,
1990), what has been called "brainstorming." In this effect, a larger
number of solutions to a problem are generated during group discussion than are generated by individuals because both individual
solutions and integrative-collective group solutions are likely to be
evoked by group discussion (Miles, 1981, pp. 119-120).

Sussman et al. (1991) investigated whether an extended focus
group procedure resulted in (a) a polarization of attitudes (a group
influence bias effect) or (b) a greater pool of ideas than those

generated by its members at pretest (brainstorming; a favorable group effect). A total of 233 ninth- through 12th-grade students were administered pretests, involved in focus group discussions lasting 30 minutes, comparable to other studies, and administered posttests. One classroom was randomly selected in each grade from among eight high schools (three from Illinois and five from southern California), blocked by urban/rural region, which were, in turn, randomly selected from a larger set of high schools. Of the students, 64% had tried cigarettes and 31% had tried smokeless tobacco.

Southern California and Illinois high school students were involved in a total of 31 focus groups ($n = 8$ per group, one per class) and were administered pretest and posttest questionnaires. These groups addressed the perceived utility of self-generated strategies designed to recruit adolescent tobacco users into a high-school-based tobacco use cessation clinic. Posttest-pretest differences were examined. Support was obtained for a group polarization effect, which was replicated across grades, regions, tobacco use status, and specific strategy type. Specifically, after participating in a focus group, students rated all self-generated cessation clinic recruitment strategies as more likely to be successful. They also reported that it was more likely that these strategies would lead them to join a program themselves if they were tobacco users. However, no support was obtained for the brainstorming effect. In the present context, focus groups do not appear to elicit reporting of new types of strategies, but do instill more favorable attitudes regarding self-generated solutions to a problem.

Focus Groups Are Still Useful

Barring evidence regarding methodological weaknesses and strengths, focus groups do provide practical solutions to topic issues. In the present study, the focus group data obtained were useful in generating an effective package of tobacco use cessation recruitment strategies, including use of incentives (e.g., class release time), advertising (e.g., posters, public announcements, class announcements), and notification to youth about use of cessation strategies of interest to them (e.g., social support; Burton, Sussman, Dent, et al., 1989; Graham et al., 1993). Furthermore, the data from the present study suggest that focus groups can themselves be used as a motivational strategy, although this was not their intended function. Indeed, relatively unstructured small group discussions have been used by health educators to organize and mobilize people to action (Basch, 1987). It is a principle of Socratic teaching used in adolescent prevention programs that having group members generate their own solutions leads to more commitment to the information transmitted than does a didactic teaching approach (Sussman, 1991). Use of focus-like groups prior to announcing the occurrence of a cessation clinic could increase student participation through manipulation of a group polarization effect. After attending what appears to be a nondirective discussion group, students who are tobacco users may be energized to attend a cessation clinic.

Focus Groups (Round 3)

Five questions were asked in Round 3, based on other discussion material. Specifically, students were asked (a) how important it was to see someone with a tobacco-related disease, (b) whether they preferred use of live or videotaped persons, (c) how important it was to use self-help materials, (d) what was the best time of day to have a group, and (e) how relevant it was to deal with drugs aside from tobacco. A total of eight groups were run in California, each composed of one classroom from each grade from each of two schools. Responses were consistent across groups. Students liked the idea of using live speakers with a disease, did not like self-help materials except for brief summary material, wanted to meet during the school day, and were mixed about dealing with other drugs. Generally, students reported feeling positive about meeting in groups but also reported that groups dealing with different drugs should meet separately so that those who just smoke won't feel stigmatized and be scared away.

Large-Scale Assessment Data

Reasons for Using and Quitting

These data are reported from 11 high schools at the southern California site. One class from each grade level at each school was surveyed; this resulted in approximately 1,000 students. Lifetime use, current use, and intentions to use cigarettes were most highly correlated with feeling good from smoking (rs = about .40), relaxation (rs = about .40), improved concentration (rs = about .35), and having something to do when bored (rs = about .33). Smoking to be popular was not significantly related to use. Reasons for smoking among adolescents were pretty much the same as with adults.

Directed to smokeless tobacco use, these same type of behavioral self-report measures were most highly correlated with taste (rs = about .35), being better than cigarettes (rs = about .27), helping with concentration (rs = about .23), something to do (rs = about .22), and with relaxation, fun, buzz, or "feels good" items (rs = about .20). Being cool or popular generally was not related to use. Smokeless tobacco reasons were similar to the cigarette reasons, except that taste and "better than cigarettes" responses were obtained. As with results of the Round 1 focus groups, the reasons for quitting tended to be normative and informational social influence oriented, or related to physical consequences. In the large-scale data, addiction was not mentioned as a reason to quit (see Table 10.1).

Stages of Cessation

A sample of 1,380 high school students from the large-scale survey in southern California in 1991 was asked to "circle the one item which describes you the best." The response choices consisted of "I've never thought about quitting," "I've thought about quitting, but haven't made up my mind," "I plan to quit right away," "I plan to quit, but not until later," "I've quit and I'm trying to stay off," and "I've thought about quitting and decided I don't want to." The question was asked twice. The first time, subjects were instructed to complete the question "only if you currently smoke cigarettes." The second time, subjects were asked to com-

Table 10.1 Most Popular Reasons for Quitting Cigarette Smoking and Smokeless Tobacco

Reason	N (%)
Smoking	293 (100)
If my girlfriend/boyfriend asked me to quit	160 (54.6)
If someone close to me died because of smoking	147 (50.2)
To live longer	143 (48.8)
If a doctor told me to quit	120 (41)
To look more attractive	99 (33.8)
Smokeless Tobacco	82 (100)
If my girlfriend/boyfriend asked me to quit	33 (40.2)
If someone close to be died because of smokeless tobacco use	33 (40.2)
To smell better	30 (36.6)
If a doctor told me to quit	24 (29.3)
To live longer	20 (24.4)
To make my folks happy	20 (24.4)

plete the question "only if you currently use chewing tobacco or snuff." According to these data, approximately 27% of the smokers and 20% of the smokeless tobacco users were thinking of quitting or wanted to quit right away. An additional 25% of smokers and smokeless tobacco users were trying to stay nonsmokers. Thus cessation clinic programming was relevant to at least half of the tobacco users (see Table 10.2).

Pilot Motivational Recruitment Study

The next phase of cessation clinic development involved the completion of a cessation clinic recruitment study that contrasted a personal power condition (emphasizing recruitment through an emphasis on themes of independence and power over tobacco use), a fear-arousal condition (emphasizing recruitment through an emphasis on a theme of fear regarding consequences of tobacco use), and a minimal information condition that merely indicated clinic availability. One-session clinics were developed and implemented at separate high schools. Two schools were randomly assigned to each condition within each site (total $N = 6$ schools in

Table 10.2   Frequency and Percentage of Smokers and Smokeless
Tobacco Users at the Different Stages of Cessation (1991)

Stage	Smokers N (%)	ST Users N (%)
I never thought about quitting.	50 (17.1)	28 (25.7)
I've thought about quitting, but haven't made up my mind.	56 (19.2)	10 (9.2)
I plan to quit right away.	22 (7.5)	12 (11.0)
I plan to quit, but not until later.	50 (17.1)	10 (9.2)
I've quit and I'm trying to stay off.	78 (26.7)	30 (27.5)
I've thought about quitting and decided I don't want to.	36 (12.4)	19 (17.4)
Total	292 (100)	109 (100)

California and total $N = 6$ schools in Illinois). Each clinic was pre-
ceded by use of a speaker (the ex-"Winston man" Dave Goerlitz),
public announcements, and flyers that were theoretically linked
to condition. For example, content of the "Winston Man's" speech
varied by condition and either emphasized personal power, emphasized fear of consequences, or only briefly summarized previous
experiences related to tobacco advertisements. In all three conditions, youth were invited to attend a one-session clinic. No differences between conditions were found. *Class release time* was the
most important incentive for clinic attendance. Without class release time, an average of 10 students had previously been found
to attend a clinic session; with class release time 50 or more
students would attend.

CESSATION CLINIC CONTENTS DEVELOPMENT

The objectives of the 1989-1990 year (Year 3) for the TNT cessation component were (a) to develop and pilot cessation clinics, and
(b) to select the most promising clinics for testing in the randomized trial to take place in 1990-1991 (Year 4). Almost all of the
piloting took place in Illinois. Six of the original 12 Illinois schools
participated in the clinic piloting—the same 6 schools that had
participated in the 1988-1989 (Year 2) motivation activities. Pilot

clinics were developed, based on separate stages of a stage model of the acquisition of dependency on tobacco (Burton, Sussman, Dent, et al., 1989; discussed earlier in this chapter), which posits that the acquisition of dependency moves through four stages: (a) social influences, (b) addiction, (c) psychosocial dependency, and (d) negative affect. Stages 1, 3, and 4 were merged into one comprehensive clinic for piloting. An addiction-focused clinic also was developed and piloted both in Illinois and in southern California. A large number of process and administrative details were addressed; the main findings and decisions based on the pilot-testing experiences are summarized below.

1. Clinics in the Year 4 trial were to be five sessions long with one additional follow-up session. Four sessions were inadequate, but some school personnel balked at having more than five sessions.
2. Clinics needed to begin with a maximum of 10 students. Students were inhibited by larger groups.
3. Clinics were to take place during class periods, staggered so that students did not miss more than one session of any regular school class.
4. Clinics were to be limited to users only, instead of users and helpers.
5. It was necessary for students to sign up in advance to participate, in a manner that provided as much confidentiality as possible (e.g., use of sign-up sheets in the nurse's office and "yellow slips" that let smokers be released from class without specifying release to the clinic).
6. Groups with female and male participants worked well as long as there was not too much of an imbalance in numbers. Overall, in Year 3, there were almost as many boys as girls participating. For the randomized trial the next year, we distributed (blocked) volunteers by gender to clinics to keep them balanced.
7. Over two-thirds of the participants in the pilot clinics cut down on their tobacco use, and there was a large, significant shift in intentions among users, with greater expectations that they would not be using tobacco one year later. However, only a small percentage of the students quit during the clinic. The foci for the last pilot groups were to decrease attrition and increase cessation during the clinics. Spacing of clinic sessions was important in minimizing attrition (two sessions in the 1st week, one session in a 2nd week, one session in a 3rd week, one session in a 5th week, and one session 3 months later.

8. It is possible that the "Addiction Only" clinic is more efficacious with smokeless tobacco users, and the "Psychosocial Dependency" clinic is more efficacious with smokers. These two clinics were refined for testing in the Year 4 randomized trial of 24 schools in Illinois and southern California (as opposed to development of a comprehensive clinic, which would counteract all four functions).

9. Successful cessation clinic recruitment was established at both sites by use of posters, public announcements (over the PA system), flyers, and use of class release time as an incentive. We learned also that face-to-face recruitment at lunchtime the day before the first clinic was to be held was a sure way to reach the maximum clinic size. Use of a speaker was *not* necessary, and it takes effort to provide an effective speaker (as had been accomplished in the recruitment study); thus speakers were not used as part of clinic recruitment.

10. Cessation curricula development went through five iterations to (a) develop and pilot test clinics, and (b) select the most promising clinic types for testing in a randomized trial in Year 4 of the grant. The pilot testing resulted in two five-session clinic programs, the one a single-component addiction-based program and the other a single-component psychosocial-based program involving social influences, psychosocial dependency, and negative affect management components (instead of being a comprehensive program; addiction material was minimized). Pilot five-session clinics were administered at both sites.

Summary of Final Cessation Program

Clinics involved eight schools at each site; within-school control groups were established based on sign-up sheets; four other schools within each site were included as no-treatment controls. Three-month follow-up data were collected at a sixth session. Self-help cessation intervention packages were provided to treatment and control school volunteers in Year 5.

Students in both conditions received a motivational audiotape written specifically for their condition in the two program conditions. They also received a quit package that included a canister of mint snuff, a cinnamon stick, a pocket calendar, and a TNT key chain. Tobacco users in both conditions received folders of quit materials.

In the *psychosocial folder*, there were five one-page handouts, which were reminders to the tobacco users regarding clinic goals. The first prepared the youth to quit tobacco. The second emphasized healing and quitting. The third emphasized coping skills. The fourth emphasized points of assertiveness and staying a nonsmoker. Finally, the fifth emphasized quit maintenance strategies including social support and reminded the youth about a 3-month reunion.

A second part of the folder included a reprint of the *Reader's Digest* article about Sean Marsee's death, which has been attributed to use of smokeless tobacco (Fincher, 1985). A third part consisted of appendix-type material, including five pages of facts on tobacco use consequences (general consequences, passive smoking, physiological details), a two-page handout on withdrawal symptoms, and a two-page handout on a floating relaxation exercise.

A third part of the folder included a 14-page cessation clinic outline that led the youth through the five clinic sessions. A summary of clinic contents is shown in Appendix F.

In the *addiction folder*, there were also five one-page handouts, which were reminders to the tobacco users regarding clinic goals. The first three were very similar to those distributed in the psychosocial program (e.g., the first prepared the youth to quit tobacco), but each handout emphasized conquering nicotine addiction as opposed to conquering psychosocial dependency to tobacco use. The fourth focused on avoidance of weight gain, and did *not* mention assertiveness. Finally, the fifth emphasized substitute behavior for one's daily routine, *not* seeking social support. Otherwise the last two handouts were similar across conditions.

The second and third part of the folder were identical to those parts in the psychosocial condition. An outline of the addiction clinic contents is shown in Appendix G.

ELEVEN

Cessation Clinic Evaluation

This chapter presents the 3-month outcomes of the cessation study. Methodological issues and controls, clinic results, and school-wide trends are discussed.

METHODOLOGICAL CONSIDERATIONS

Many of the general methodological considerations for cessation were the same as those for prevention, as outlined in Chapters 5 and 6. These considerations include concerns of biochemical validation and other corroborative measures, sample selection and assignment, and attrition. However, at least four cessation-specific considerations deserve mention:

1. The means of selection differ between classroom-based prevention and clinic-based cessation programming. Youth in prevention programming are a "captive audience" of such programming; most youths in the school would be exposed to it and would be evaluated. With cessation, on the other hand, only those youth who are recruited to the clinic program would be evaluated. Thus subject selection is a greater problem.

2. Length of follow-up is an issue that differentiates prevention from cessation programming. In prevention programming, effects on behavior usually do not occur for at least one year postprogram for a 7th-grade cohort (although some anecdotal reports suggest that

smoking onset changes can be detected over a 3-month pre-post summer interval). In cessation programming, effects on behavior occur immediately and relapse is a focal issue. The follow-up interval to assess relapse often is completed beginning at 3 months postprogram, although among adults a period of at least one year is preferable (Glasgow & Lichtenstein, 1987; Lichtenstein & Glasgow, 1992; Lichtenstein & Mermelstein, 1984). Among adolescents, determining an adequate follow-up period is complicated by the issue of the rather dynamic nature of smoking in adolescence (Pallonen et al., 1990). Of course, defining cessation (e.g., cumulative prevalence, point prevalence) is an issue with both adolescents and adults (Lichtenstein & Glasgow, 1992; Lichtenstein & Mermelstein, 1984; Pallonen et al., 1990; Velicer, Prochaska, Rossi, & Snow, 1992).

3. Attrition also becomes a different issue in a cessation program compared to a prevention program. In prevention trials, all subjects receive the program, and follow-up is completed on at least 70% of the sample. In cessation programming, on the other hand, approximately half of the subjects will drop out after an initial meeting (among adults; e.g., Sussman, Whitney-Saltiel, et al., 1989). Efforts are needed to maintain attendance at most or all clinic sessions. Only half of clinic attenders usually will attend an aftercare session, if offered. Finally, those who do not quit tobacco use may not be interested in participating in follow-up activities.

4. Replicability of results may be more of an issue in cessation than in prevention programming. As summarized by Lichtenstein and Mermelstein (1984), small sample sizes (also see section on statistical power later in this chapter), different means of recruitment, and relatively high variability in eventual outcomes within each group (particularly among adolescents) make replicability a major issue to grapple with in the design of a cessation program.

In Project TNT, we handled each of these four cessation-specific methodological issues as described in the last chapter or in detail below. We dealt with selection concerns by developing a means of recruiting subjects that would motivate a majority, or at least a large number, of smokers to sign up on a cessation clinic waiting list (i.e., use of school release time). Second, we used a 3-month follow-up period to assess cessation, which appears adequate with adolescents, who change behavior more rapidly than adults. Third, we calculated outcomes not controlling for, and controlling for, effects of attrition. Assuming that those who do not show up at follow-up are still using tobacco is a conservative means of calculating cessation (Lichtenstein & Mermelstein, 1984). Finally, we dealt with selection and replicability concerns by randomly assigning subjects from the waiting lists to conditions, including subjects from two regions of the country, and measuring school-wide trends—realizing that subject selection and replicability remain basic issues in all tobacco use cessation clinic research (Lichtenstein & Glasgow, 1992).

Design of Randomized Cessation Trial

A 20-page questionnaire was administered to the 24 participating high schools: 12 high schools in California and 12 in Illinois, half rural and half urban/suburban in each case. A longitudinal trend design was used for 3 years, 1988, 1990, and 1991 (Years 2, 4, and 5 of the project). In California one class and in Illinois two classes were randomly selected from all of the general track classes at each grade level for survey administration during the fall of the respective school years.

The 24 schools were randomly assigned, within state and region (rural versus suburban), to three conditions: (a) addiction clinics, (b) psychosocial dependency clinics, and (c) no clinics. Within each of the 16 treatment schools, students volunteering to participate in a cessation clinic were randomly assigned to be in a clinic or were instructed that the clinics were filled. Two clinics were held at each of the treatment schools (the same type of clinic within school). The clinics consisted of five sessions spaced over a 1-month period. The sixth follow-up session was held 3 months after the fifth session; students who had volunteered for the clinics but been randomized to the control condition were also invited to the "3-month" follow-up session. At the follow-up session, students were asked to indicate (verbally) whether they had completely quit all tobacco use. Those subjects reporting cessation were then administered a saliva test, which was analyzed. All subjects were then administered the written follow-up questionnaire. (Subsequent to the study, students at all participating schools were offered self-help tobacco use cessation materials free of charge.)

This overall design makes it possible to assess (a) the efficacy of clinics versus no clinics (students admitted to clinics versus those not admitted within each of the 16 treatment schools), (b) the relative efficacy of the addiction versus the psychosocial dependency clinics (participants in the addiction clinics in eight of the treatment schools versus those in the psychosocial clinics in the other eight treatment schools), and (c) the extent of any generalization of treatment effects to other students in the school (changes in survey data from 1990 to 1991 in the 16 treatment schools versus the eight control schools).

Statistical Power

Power could not be calculated for the cessation studies because we knew of no data upon which effect size calculations could be based, and the area is very underresearched. However, all analyses using the individual as the unit had approximately 70 subjects per condition, so statistical power was more than adequate even for the most fine-grained analysis.

RESULTS OF RANDOMIZED CESSATION TRIAL

Preintervention School-Wide Trends

Preintervention trends can be examined through the 1988 and 1990 surveys. (The intervention began in 1990 after the surveys had been administered.) In the 12 Illinois schools, weekly smoking or greater among boys increased from 22.5% in 1988 to 26.4% in 1990; among girls there was a decrease from 29.3% in 1988 to 27.2% in 1990. Among Illinois boys, smokeless tobacco use decreased from 18.1% to 13.2% in the 12 schools. However, all of this decrease in smokeless tobacco use took place in the 6 suburban schools, where use went from 29.2% in 1988 to 10.9% in 1990. In the rural schools, smokeless tobacco use doubled, going from 8.5% to 16.2%. In California, smoking among boys decreased from 23.0% in 1988 to 18.1% in 1990, and among girls it decreased from 25.3% to 18.9%. Smokeless tobacco use among boys decreased from 8.5% to 5.9% (reflecting decreases at both rural and suburban schools).

Cessation Clinic Results

For the 16 treatment schools (8 in California and 8 in Illinois) there was a 48.4% attrition during the clinic from Session 1 to Session 5. All of the cessation results reported here are calculated in the most conservative way, using all students who came to the first clinic session as the denominator; thus all of the students who did not come to the fifth session were assumed to be using tobacco, regardless of how many previous sessions they had attended.

There were significant differences in smoking cessation by clinic model, with 25.7% of those in the psychosocial dependency clinics compared with 10.5% of those in the addiction clinics reporting end-of-clinic cessation, based on a total of 184 students who were smokers only. There were no statistically significant differences for the 42 smokeless tobacco users, although the results appear to be in the opposite direction, with 35.3% of those in the addiction clinics compared with 24.0% of those in the psychosocial dependency clinics reporting end-of-clinic cessation. Similarly, of the 18 students who both smoked and used smokeless tobacco, 50.0% in the addiction clinics and 33.3% in the psychosocial dependency clinics reported end-of-clinic cessation of both substances.

There was an additional 60.6% attrition between the end of the clinic (fifth session) and the 3-month follow-up (sixth session). If we consider only those students who came for the 3-month follow-up as our denominator, we find that 19.8% of the smokers who had participated in clinics, compared with 10.5% of those who had not been admitted to clinics, reported quitting smoking; 43.8% of the 16 smokeless tobacco users who had participated in clinics reported quitting, compared with 0% of the five smokeless tobacco control subjects. However, when we apply the conservative interpretation to the results and use all students who had volunteered to participate in the clinic as the denominator, we find that 8.4%

Table 11.1 Tobacco Use Cessation Clinic Results Collapsed Across Illinois and California

	Clinic Attenders	*Wait List*
Those who attended the 3-month follow-up		
Percent quit smoking	19.8	10.5
Percent quit smokeless tobacco use	43.8	0.0
Total sample: included those students who attended Session 1 and dropped out		
Percent quit smoking	8.4	10.5
Percent quit smokeless tobacco use	17.4	0.0
Total sample: also corrected by biochemical validation		
Percent quit smoking	6.8	7.9
Percent quit smokeless tobacco use	15.2	0.0
Total sample: also corrected by biochemical validation and written questionnaire responses		
Percent quit smoking	4.2	7.9
Percent quit smokeless tobacco use	13.0	0.0

NOTE: Smokers only, $n = 184$; smokeless tobacco users only, $n = 42$; both smokers and smokeless tobacco users, $n = 18$; total $N = 244$ clinic participants.

of the smokers who had participated in clinics and 10.5% of the control subjects reported quitting all tobacco use, and 17.4% of the smokeless tobacco users who had participated in the clinics compared with 0% of the control subjects reported quitting. Moreover, when results are corrected by biochemical results (using saliva cotinine for validation), the 3-month cessation results for confirmed tobacco cessation are 6.8% for clinic participants and 7.9% for control subjects who had been smokers, and 15.2% versus 0% for clinic versus control subjects who had been smokeless tobacco users. Finally, when we look at the results for subjects who were biochemically confirmed as quitting and who indicated on the written questionnaire that they had quit, we find that only 4.2% of the clinic participants and 7.9% of the control subjects who had been smokers had quit, whereas 13% of the clinic participants and none of the control subjects who had been smokeless tobacco users quit. The results are shown in Table 11.1.

Pre- to Postintervention School-Wide Trends

Across all 12 schools in Illinois, smoking remained about the same between 1990 and 1991 for both boys (26.4% and 27.6%) and girls (27.2% and 26.7%). The trends for rural and suburban schools were consistent for boys. However, smoking among girls increased in rural schools (from 25.6.% to 29.2%) and decreased in suburban schools (28.3% to 24.5%). Similarly, in Illinois, smokeless tobacco use among boys stayed about the same (13.2% and 12.8%), with no differences in trends between rural and suburban schools. In the 12 California schools, smoking increased from 18.1% to 24.6% among boys, and from 18.9% to 24.8% among girls, with no differences in direction of trends between rural and suburban schools. Similarly, smokeless tobacco use increased among boys in California from 5.9% to 9.1%, reflecting increases in both rural and suburban schools.

Even though schools were randomly assigned to conditions, tobacco use at baseline was somewhat higher at the treatment schools than the control school. Still, school-wide trends from before to after the clinic period could be examined to assess the degree to which cessation clinics either influenced school-wide trends or simply reflected school-wide trends. In the California schools, tobacco use increased in both the treatment and control schools. Smoking increased from 20.8% to 27.2% in the treatment schools and from 14.1% to 20.8% in the control schools. Smokeless tobacco use among boys increased from 6.7% to 11.2% in the treatment schools and from 4.5% to 6.0% in the control schools. In the Illinois schools smoking decreased slightly from 27.1% to 25.4% in the treatment schools and increased from 26.2% to 30.7% in the control schools. Smokeless tobacco use among boys stayed about the same in the treatment schools (15.1% and 15.5%) and decreased in the control schools from 9.0% to 7.8%. Thus clinic activities neither influenced nor were influenced by school-wide trends.

PART FIVE

Conclusions and Future Directions in Tobacco Use Prevention and Cessation Programs

Part Five, the final section, presents conclusions based on Project TNT prevention and cessation programming, and suggests future directions for tobacco use prevention and cessation research and practice. Chapter 12 discusses implications of the results of the Project TNT prevention and cessation studies. Finally, Chapter 13 discusses remaining general issues in adolescent tobacco use research.

TWELVE

Discussion of Prevention and Cessation Results

This chapter first discusses how one might interpret the results obtained in the prevention study. It then discusses the issue of providing school-based smokeless tobacco prevention programming to both boys and girls when boys are its main users. Finally, it interprets the cessation clinic results.

INTERPRETATION OF PREVENTION RESULTS

These data from the prevention program suggest that (a) physical consequences information can be used to compose a curriculum that is as successful as a social influence program, (b) a normative social influence program is not as efficacious for tobacco use prevention as are other types of programs, except for prevention of smokeless tobacco onset at the 1-year follow-up or onset of cigarette smoking at the 2-year follow-up, and (c) the same tobacco use prevention programming can be successful when targeted on both use of cigarettes and smokeless tobacco in the school-based context (see Sussman, Dent, Stacy, Sun, et al., 1993; Dent et al., 1994).

The physical consequences condition was as efficacious as the social influence programs in most comparisons. This pattern of results may contradict previous research, which found that social influence programming is more successful than physical consequences programming. On the other hand, the present physical consequences curriculum included several novel features, such as correcting myths about tobacco experimentation and addiction, role-playing diseases, and presenting probabilities of consequences information in ways more personally relevant to youth. Previous physical consequences curricula focused more on didactic instruction of long-term consequences information. Although generally not measured in previous studies, social influence prevention programming may have been more successful in earlier studies due to being better received by students than traditional approaches.

The data regarding the normative social influence condition suggest that teaching refusal assertion skills and classmate peer disapproval of tobacco use was ineffective in this sample (aside from prevention of trial of smokeless tobacco at the 1-year follow-up or trial of smoking at the 2-year follow-up). A previous analysis has revealed that process ratings were slightly lower in this condition. Anecdotally, health educators and students reported that the "flooding" of their school systems and homes with normative social influence programs (e.g., red ribbon week, "Just Say No" campaign public service announcements) may have led to lack of excitement over additional normative social influence information. This lack of enthusiasm due to familiarity with normative social influence material may have affected the results obtained. Nonetheless, knowledge items in the survey indicated that students in the normative social influence condition learned more about this type of information than did students in the other conditions. Thus there is no ceiling effect on their learning of this type of information.

Another possibility is that the apparent effectiveness of refusal assertion skills training, the main normative social influence component in previous smoking prevention programs, may have been due to the confounding or interaction of training in refusal assertion skills with other social influence program components. Most social influence programs that have taught refusal assertion skills also have taught some aspects of informational social influence. In the present project, the informational social influence condition exerted stronger overall effects than the normative social influence condition on smoking, which is consistent with this interpretation. The stronger overall effects of the informational social influence condition over the normative social influence condition may imply that teaching students how to more effectively interpret social sources of information is more important than teaching specific refusal assertion skills (or facts about classroom levels of peer disapproval for using tobacco products).

Another way of interpreting social influence condition effects is by observing the pattern of differences in effects obtained between the normative and informational social influence conditions at 1 or 2 years postprogram. At the 1-year follow-up, the informational social influence condition had exerted an effect on cigarette smoking but not on smokeless tobacco use, and the normative social influence condition had exerted an effect on smokeless tobacco use (trial behavior) but not on cigarette smoking. This finding converges with some pilot study data that indicated effects of refusal assertion training on intention to use smokeless tobacco but not on intention to smoke cigarettes. One may conjecture that teaching refusal assertion skills is effective for prevention of trying smokeless tobacco because normative social influence pressures are more prevalent for use of this substance (e.g., related to dares to use a new substance), whereas informational social influence pressures (e.g., magazine advertising) are more prevalent for cigarettes. Alternatively, perhaps simply learning that one should say no to offers of smokeless tobacco is perceived as novel to adolescents, whereas the same instruction is perceived as being "nothing new" regarding cigarettes.

Still, at 2-year follow-up (9th grade), the normative and informational social influence conditions showed the same effects on prevalence of tobacco use from immediate posttest. It apparently is the case that either single-component program is only effective on trial of smoking in the long run. Possibly normative social influence becomes a more important fact to counteract as youth reach high school (see discussion on changing patterns of social influences in the school in Chapter 13). Perhaps both social influences programs were effectively counteracting two sources of social influence that now were of equal valence in facilitating trial of smoking. In any case, their combined effects are needed to have an impact on higher levels of use of smoking or smokeless tobacco.

The combined condition was the most efficacious at 1-year follow-up. This condition was the only one that showed a preventive effect on weekly use of smokeless tobacco as well as on the other three behavioral outcomes at the 1-year follow-up. We did not expect to achieve a relative superiority of the combined condition. As reported previously, greater teaching effort was required to impart this thematically diverse material. Also, modification of curriculum material during implementation was relatively likely, possibly the result of attempts to provide a theoretical integration of the different perspectives. Finally, knowledge learned from the combined curriculum was relatively likely to be diluted. In other words, students were likely to learn less about more material. Although each of these effects of a heterogeneous curriculum conceivably could have detrimental effects on program success, the heterogeneity of the combined curriculum instead led to the strongest overall effects at the 1-year follow-up. At the 2-year follow-up, the combined condition and the physical consequences condition showed a differential impact on use of the two tobacco products.

The overall predictive superiority of the combined condition at 1 year might imply that different causes of tobacco use need to be counteracted simultaneously because the behavior is determined by multiple causes. Also, a heterogeneous program may reach a wider variety of youth who may differ in risk factors that influence use. One might conclude that current comprehensive social influence programming should be continued and emphasized over the development of isolated program components. On the other hand, at 2 years, although it was the only curriculum to affect weekly cigarette smoking, the physical consequences curriculum was the only one to affect trial of smokeless tobacco use. As youth grew older, they remembered the Sean Marsee memorial lesson from the physical consequences curriculum better than from the combined curriculum, which may have led to the relatively strong effects on smokeless tobacco use in that condition. Identification with a high school peer who died from smokeless tobacco use may have had an impact on youth through personal identification with the victim (as discussed in Chapter 4).

Summary of Prevention Results and Conclusions

The results of this project at 1-year follow-up indicated that activities designed to counteract normative social influence were effective only in the prevention of trial of smokeless tobacco; activities designed to counteract informational social influence were effective in the prevention of trial and weekly cigarette smoking; activities designed to counteract physical consequences misperceptions were effective in prevention of trial of both cigarettes and smokeless tobacco, and of weekly cigarette smoking, but not of weekly smokeless tobacco use. The combined condition was effective in the prevention of all four outcome behaviors. By the 2-year follow-up, all conditions showed effects on trial use of cigarettes; the physical consequences condition showed effects on trial and weekly use of smokeless tobacco; and the combined condition showed effects on weekly cigarette smoking and weekly smokeless tobacco use. Only the physical consequences condition affected trial of smokeless tobacco use, and only the combined condition affected weekly cigarette use. The difference in the pattern of results from immediate posttest to 8th grade, versus from immediate posttest to 9th grade, is quite interesting. Although the two strongest curricula at 1-year follow-up remained the strongest curricula at 2-year follow-up, their effects on tobacco differed somewhat between time points. In the long run, physical consequences information was especially important for the prevention of smokeless tobacco use. A modified combined condition that adds a little more physical consequences information is likely to remain the strongest and most generalized program overall.

DELIVERY OF CLASSROOM-BASED TOBACCO USE PREVENTION: ALL PRODUCTS?

Of current concern in tobacco use prevention research is the determination of whether information targeting smokeless tobacco use and cigarette smoking should be presented alone or together. If information was provided on smokeless tobacco alone, the program would be more focused. However, in various contexts (e.g., school-based programs), smokeless-tobacco-only education would be of little use to the female subjects. Thus, for this pragmatic reason, prevention programming for both cigarettes and smokeless tobacco may be needed. In addition, there are several advantages to delivering smokeless tobacco prevention programming in combination with smoking prevention material. First, the combined approach would be relevant to a larger proportion of the population than either would separately (e.g., males who primarily smoke cigarettes). Second, with the exception of product information, physical consequences information, and consideration of the more restricted contexts of smokeless tobacco use (e.g., among high-risk males), the contents of the two programs are likely to be very similar and complement one another. Social influence strategies, for example, tend to have an impact on use of both substances. Finally, if either program was delivered exclusive of the other, there might be a tendency for the subjects to assume that the other form of tobacco was safe. Programs that solely emphasize the risks, teach correct prevalence estimates, and provide mechanisms for avoiding smoking, for example, may be construed by participants as condoning smokeless tobacco use.

Project TNT developed and provided curricula that address both substances. Each curriculum contained a nearly identical percentage of references made to each tobacco product. In the combined curriculum, for example, across all 10 lessons the percentage of references made to each tobacco product was as follows: smokeless tobacco (22%), pipes (3%), cigars (3%), cigarettes or smoking (65%), and "tobacco products" as a generic reference (7%). In other words, approximately one fourth of tobacco product information addressed smokeless tobacco and two thirds addressed cigarettes.

INTERPRETATION OF CESSATION RESULTS

The clinic results must be interpreted in light of concurrently static or increasing school-wide trends of tobacco use during that period that might tend to deflate results obtained. Also, attrition was as high as in adult programs. Results therefore need to be interpreted with some caution.

The data suggested that addiction was a more important concern for smokeless tobacco than for cigarettes. Smokeless tobacco users showed a higher quit rate than smokers in the addiction clinics (though not significantly so), whereas the converse result was found in the psychosocial dependency clinic condition. This result trend is consistent with some of the literature indicating higher blood nicotine levels among smokeless tobacco users than smokers (U.S. DHHS, 1989). The topography of use also suggests that craving is a more major problem with smokeless tobacco use than with smoking (U.S. DHHS, 1994). One dip of snuff has the same level of nicotine as three to four cigarettes. A person who takes a dip once every 30 minutes is like a smoker who chain smokes four cigarettes over that same period. Coping with cravings, not surprisingly, becomes important very soon in the life of a smokeless tobacco user (Ary et al., 1989).

The psychosocial dependency clinics were relatively successful for cigarettes. This result is not surprising because social influences are likely to operate throughout high school (as discussed in the next chapter of this book) and are likely to be related to psychosocial dependency needs (e.g., to reduce loneliness). Psychosocial dependency functions tend not to be incorporated in many prevention programs (cf. Wills, 1986). Perhaps the individualized meanings of cigarette smoking as an ego-enhancing device for smokers are of more importance once social influence information is internalized by the tobacco user. At the point when solitary smoking becomes more of an issue, which does occur during high school (Sussman, Hahn, et al., 1993; also see Chapter 6 of this book), psychosocial dependency becomes of real importance. Thus it is of relevance to consider material counteracting psychosocial dependency in the development of future adolescent smoking cessation programming. Consideration of alternative means of developing higher self-esteem and one's desired identity (e.g., as an "individual"; Burton, Sussman, Hansen, et al., 1989) such as alternative, prosocial behavior (e.g., engaging in a unique hobby) or prosocial coping with stresses (e.g., seeking spiritual support, seeking social support, relaxation; Wills, 1986), needs to be incorporated into such programming.

When statistical adjustments to tobacco use cessation rates were placed on the data, as discussed in the last chapter, cessation rates decreased among those in the clinic conditions. Combined across clinics, as shown earlier in Table 11.1, smoking rates decreased from 20% to 4%, and smokeless tobacco use cessation rates decreased from 44% to 13%. When compared to the wait list controls (matched on motivation to quit), rates of quitting smoking were much higher for clinic attendees before adjustments were made, but were only higher for smokeless tobacco users after adjustments were made. In particular, the clinic dropout adjustment accounted for the dissipation of the smoking cessation results. Future research demands the following up of dropouts to see if they are, indeed, still smoking. Corroborative data from clinic attendees and follow-up of a subsample of dropouts did indicate that indeed all 100% of dropouts were still smoking. Cost considerations kept us from completing an exhaustive follow-up. The results, conservatively examined, suggest that the clinic works for those who do attend it and "work it." Smokers who are motivated to quit may need a clinic and relevant information to help them quit. Smokeless tobacco use cessation, on the other hand, appears to occur *only* if there is a clinic provided (although the sample size was small).

Also, we should mention that more work needs completion regarding the Burton, Sussman, Dent, et al. (1989) model. Though this model is theoretically appealing, empirical support for four functionally separable stages is lacking. We recently completed a crosssectional structural modeling analysis (not reported elsewhere in this book) separately for smokers and smokeless tobacco users, using a "dependency scale" that was created by our research team (Burton et al., 1994). The data used were from the Illinois high school survey in Year 2 ($n = 240$). Three items were created for each of the four hypothesized stages of adolescent tobacco use: social influence, addiction, psychosocial dependency, and negative affect. The results indicated two fairly strong factors describing smokers but only one factor describing smokeless tobacco users. What we had labeled psychosocial dependency and addiction loaded on the same factor (which one might refer to as "addictive dependency," incorporating both physiological and psychological components). The second factor was composed of social influence and negative affect stages. This finding was surprising, for we had theorized that these two stages were not adjacent ones, but rather that negative affect was the last stage and social influence was the first stage. One might refer to this second factor as "reactive dependency": that is, reacting to social or intrapsychic pressures by smoking.

These results suggest that use of smokeless tobacco among adolescents is unidimensional, whereas smoking is bidimensional. Thus tailoring programming to two types of smokers may need consideration within a comprehensive cessation program, whereas a conceptually integrated comprehensive program may be most effective for smokeless tobacco users. These results do not support a four-stage model, at least not the sequence suggested by Burton, Sussman, Dent, et al. (1989). On the other hand, the structural modeling procedure used cross-sectional data and does not provide a definitive disconfirmation of that model, which is longitudinal in conception.

In summary, the results of this, the largest tobacco use cessation trial to date for adolescents at school-based clinics (U.S. DHHS, 1994), suggest that many youths may not want to attend clinics (just like adults), but that cessation rates are not much lower than with adults. The clinics consisted of only six sessions and some self-help material. Cessation rates were higher than for many minimal interventions with adults (e.g., Flay, 1987b; Lichtenstein & Glasgow, 1992). The future of tobacco use cessation among adolescents is not hopeless; more research is needed. In particular, there needs to be a means to (a) maintain student involvement in all clinic sessions (consider school health education course credits) and (b) encourage students to quit now rather than when they are older. The latter need can be addressed, perhaps, by adding material mentioned in the physical-consequences-oriented prevention program (Glynn et al., 1985). If youth know that the longer they smoke, the more damage they endure, perhaps they may want to quit sooner.

For current practitioners, we recommend the following construction of tobacco cessation clinics. Just as with school-based prevention, both males and females and both smokers and smokeless tobacco users should be included in the same intervention groups at school-based cessation clinics. Probably three fourths of the material should pertain to cigarette smoking, and other material can refer to generic use of tobacco products or smokeless tobacco, to reflect relative prevalence of different types of users in the clinics. Also, considering both products and genders, it is likely that a combined condition cessation program, just as with prevention, is likely to be most successful (e.g., Sussman, Dent, Stacy, Sun, et al., 1993).

Psychosocial dependency needs certainly apply to both products, especially for those who have used long enough to internalize images associated with tobacco use. Likewise, approximately 25% of adolescent smokers and 50% of adolescent smokeless tobacco users will report craving (e.g., Ary et al., 1989; Sussman, Dent, Stacy, et al., 1989), although at least one study has not found a relation between number of cigarettes smoked (one measure of addiction) and self-initiated cessation (Hansen, Collins, Johnson, & Graham, 1985). In Project TNT, even though we were careful to keep clinic contents separate, how to deal with withdrawal symptoms needed passing mention in both types of clinics. Thus we recommend that a combined clinic be used in future programming, and we further suggest that three fourths of a clinic be psychosocial dependency based and one fourth be addiction based. We believe this relative percentage of the types of material as clinic contents reflects appropriate amount of counteraction of each type of antecedent.

THIRTEEN

Remaining General Issues in Adolescent Tobacco Use Research

This chapter discusses several remaining needs for future tobacco use prevention and cessation research, including research and programming (a) in high schools, (b) with "high-risk" youth, (c) with ethnic minorities, (d) in novel intervention contexts (e.g., by telephone), and (e) with involvement of school personnel. This chapter also discusses the need for new theoretical orientations (e.g., the memory approach). Finally, this chapter discusses the extent to which we believe school-based adolescent prevention and cessation research is advanced enough for dissemination of these programs to schools.

NEED FOR PREVENTION AND CESSATION PROGRAMMING IN HIGH SCHOOLS

Importance of Prevention Programming in High School

The need for tobacco use prevention programming among high school students is documented by two primary lines of evidence. The first line of evidence is provided by research showing that school-based prevention programs implemented in junior high school have little chance of long-term success, especially for those youth who began using tobacco before the prevention program was implemented, unless such programs are "boosted" (reviewed) or similar programming is offered possibly throughout high school (Flay et al., 1989; Murray, Pirie, Luepker, & Pallonen; 1989; Vartiainen, Pallonen, McAlister, & Puska, 1990). Prevention program effects achieved in 7th grade may be maintained through 9th or 10th grades (Flay, 1985; Flay et al., 1989; Luepker, Johnson, Murray, & Pechacek, 1983) but will dissipate by 12th grade. Of course, an initial junior high school program may be necessary to guard against the initiation of smoking in junior high school (Flay et al., 1989; Silvestri & Flay, 1989).

Additional support for the importance of high-school-based programming is provided by the dynamic social changes occurring between early adolescence (junior high school) and later adolescence (high school). At this later time point, youth spend more time away from adults, and their lives become less dominated by social interactions with small groups of same-sexed peers. Concomitantly, they become exposed to a wider range of unsupervised social gatherings that consist more of interactions with crowds, more dyadic relationships such as dating, and more "weak" ties (liaisons) than in earlier years (e.g., Dunphy, 1963; Gavin & Furman, 1989; Shrum & Cheek, 1987). Of course, social-situational factors, including same-sex peer group relationships, still remain quite important predictors of tobacco use across both junior high school and high school (Flay et al., 1983; Hahn et al., 1990; Levanthal & Cleary, 1980; McCandless & Coop, 1979; Sussman, 1989; Sussman et al., 1990). Age-appropriate high-school-based material should be provided so that youth will recall and put into practice relevant prevention strategies applicable in current high-school-aged social situations, such as jobs, team sports, and unsupervised recreational time, that provide challenges different than those experienced in earlier grades. Providing prevention programming throughout high school thus maximizes the probability that students will remain nonusers as they reach young adulthood, provided such programming takes into account the dynamic social-contextual changes characterizing this period of development.

If youth do receive prevention programming in junior high school and then are to receive booster programming in high school, it is optimal that high-school-based material can "stand on its own" (i.e., that it be provided as a minicourse). Reasons why a stand-alone program is desirable include that (a) such a program is likely to serve a thorough review function of material learned in junior high school, whereas traditional booster programs tend to provide minimal information; and (b) such a program provides assistance to students who were not previously exposed to programming (e.g., new transfers into the school district). Many students in high school only have received brief programming in junior high school (e.g., assemblies; Barovich et al., 1988; Sussman, Dent, Stacy, Sun, et al., 1993). This lack of programming is relevant not only for its public health implications but also for a study of theoretical processes of change in the operation of antecedents of tobacco use occurring from junior high school to high school, for those who have and have not received the junior high school programming.

Application of a Social Influences Prevention Curriculum to High-School-Aged Youth

Because of the desirability of providing a stand-alone high-school-based program, it is relevant to incorporate knowledge obtained from existing high-school-based prevention programs. As summarized by Flay (1987a), three high-school-based tobacco use prevention studies have published data that indicate the superiority of a comprehensive social influences program over a physical consequences program in the prevention of regular (e.g., weekly) cigarette smoking (Perry et al., 1980, 1983; Johnson, 1986; Johnson, Hansen, Collins, & Graham, 1986), though not on trying cigarettes. Also, other prevention programs using social influences curricula to target a variety of drugs of abuse have been implemented successfully with high school students (e.g., Botvin, 1986). However, there is relatively less research about social influence processes in this age group compared with younger groups, although it is known that social influences continue to operate throughout high school regarding tobacco use experimentation (e.g., Hahn et al., 1990; Sussman et al., 1990).

It is not surprising that programming would not have an effect on onset, for at least 70% of youth have already tried a cigarette by the time they reach 10th grade (e.g., Sussman, Dent, Mestel-Rauch, et al., 1988). Tentative conclusions based on these few studies suggest that comprehensive social influences prevention programming in high schools can prevent regular use. On the other hand, we have found trial use of smokeless tobacco use to increase more sharply in the 9th and 10th grades than in junior high school (from 8th to 9th grade, 15%-20%; from 9th to 10th grade, 20%-35%). Thus prevention of both trial and regular use of smokeless tobacco in high school is a possibility. Still, the relative importance of the three main social influence prevention components in high school versus junior high school is not known.

Shifts in the Relevance of Comprehensive Social Influence Components as a Function of Grade

In Project TNT, different school-based tobacco use prevention curricula were developed as a means of identifying the mediators of successful social influence programs. Curricula were designed to counteract the types of tobacco use acquisition variables typically addressed within a comprehensive social influences program: (a) peer approval for using tobacco (normative social influence), (b) incorrect social knowledge about tobacco use (informational social influence), (c) lack of knowledge about physical consequences of tobacco use, or (d) combined influences related to social and physical consequences. The literature that discusses potential grade differences in the operation of the different types of social influences and physical consequences information also addresses the potential change of importance of these influences from around 7th to 12th grades—a grade range not addressed by the current 2-year outcomes data. Changing influences across the grade range would suggest that different curricula might be relatively effective in different grades.

*Normative Versus Informational Social Influence Across Junior
High and Senior High School and Curricula Implications*

Seven studies were found that addressed changes in normative
or informational social influence as a function of junior high or
high school age. In these studies, normative social influence refers
to peer approval or direct pressure to engage in an antisocial act,
which could include to smoke or use smokeless tobacco, and
compliance behavior to this pressure. Informational social influence refers primarily to peer or adult smoking, or conformity
based on perceived correctness of others' behavior. Normative
social influence was found to increase from junior high to high
school in the four studies in which it was assessed (Berndt, 1979;
Clasen & Brown, 1985; Gavin & Furman, 1989; Salomon et al.,
1984). A slight decrease was observed by 12th grade in two studies
(Berndt, 1979; Gavin & Furman, 1989), but not in the other two
(Clasen & Brown, 1985; Salomon et al., 1984). Informational social
influence was found to increase from junior high to high school in
two of the four studies in which it was assessed (Krosnick & Judd,
1982; Salomon et al., 1984), whereas it was found to decrease in
two other studies (Costanzo & Shaw, 1966; Urberg, Cheng, &
Shyu, 1991). Informational social influence did not show a clear
pattern of increasing or decreasing by high school grade. It is
possible that normative social influence increases over grades,
whereas informational social influence perhaps becomes relatively
less important than normative social influence (e.g., Salomon et
al., 1984). This literature is interesting in that even though a
degrouping process may occur during high school (Shrum &
Cheek, 1987), pressures for misconduct increase. On the basis of
this literature, one might predict that programming developed to
counteract normative social influence would become more important during high school in larger social contexts ("crowds"; Dunphy,
1963) as well as through dyadic interactions between individuals
within or across different crowds (Shrum & Cheek, 1987). Perhaps,
as individuals grow closer in age to adulthood, their peers place
more and more direct pressure on them to give in to "dares," to
show independence, or to hurry into adultlike roles (Bachman,
O'Malley, & Johnston, 1984; Jessor, 1984; Lewis & Lewis, 1984). On

the other hand, programming developed to counteract informational social influence may become relatively less important. By high school, youth probably are well acquainted with social images associated with tobacco use, and they may more accurately ascertain reasons for tobacco advertising (Johnson et al., 1993). Still, opportunities for informational social influence regarding tobacco use abound during high school, such as through social learning mechanisms. For example, prevalence of use greatly increases. Also, although little tobacco use by students may be observed on junior high school campuses, tobacco use by students is readily observed on high school campuses (Sussman, Hahn, et al., 1993).

In summary, the importance of normative social influence on use of tobacco products is likely to be greater in high school than in junior high school. The importance of informational social influence may remain important because, although media advertisements may be more critically evaluated by high school students, more widespread opportunities for modeling effects exist in high school. It is possible that normative social influences programming will increase in preventive impact in high school, although normative plus informational social influences programming may show an even greater impact.

Physical Consequences

In Project TNT, the physical consequences condition was as effective as or more effective than the single-component social influence conditions (in junior high schools), and it was the only condition to affect trial of smokeless tobacco at the 2-year follow-up, perhaps because it contains novel features such as role-playing diseases and correcting myths about addiction (Sussman, Dent, Stacy, Hodgson, et al., 1993; Sussman, Dent, Stacy, Sun, et al., 1993). Thus a physical consequences component can be effective. If normative social influence increases in importance during high school, as a single-component curriculum it may surpass the effectiveness of the physical consequences condition. On the other hand, to the extent that physical consequences information remains important across grades, it may remain superior in preventive effect to social influence single-component material. The Flay et al. (1983) model suggests that as use increases, physiological reinforcement becomes more important. Consequently immediate and longer-term physical consequences from use may become increasingly important reasons to not use tobacco (e.g., prevention of addiction and shortness of breath).

Implications of the Combined Condition in Project TNT

Greater teaching effort was required to impart this thematically diverse material. Also, students learned less about more material in this condition (Sussman, Dent, Stacy, Hodgson, et al., 1993). Still, this condition led to the strongest overall effects at 1-year and 2-year follow-up (Sussman, Dent, Stacy, Sun, et al., 1993). In particular, this condition affected weekly cigarette smoking and smokeless tobacco use. It is possible that relatively heavy tobacco use is a function of multiple causes operating simultaneously, in which case it is possible that only a comprehensive program will affect its use. As youth enter high school, a greater variety of social (groups, crowds, romantic dyads) and activity (jobs, independent time, emphasis on team sports) situations lead to even greater variation in reasons for tobacco use. To the extent that reasons for use increase across grades, a combined condition may be relatively effective in high school. Also, by the 10th grade, weekly use of smokeless tobacco rises to 6.5% (up from 2.5% in 8th grade). Thus a replication study of the results achieved in junior high school with a larger group of users is available at the high school level.

Relevance of Classroom-Based Cessation Programming

In addition to providing prevention information, some cessation-oriented programming would be relevant to include in a program that extends into later high school. In Project TNT high schools, approximately 12% of 9th graders, 15% of 10th graders, 18% of 11th graders, and 21% of 12th graders are weekly (or more frequent) users of tobacco products. Approximately an equal percentage of nonusers are close friends of these regular tobacco users. Furthermore, twice the percentage of weekly smokers have smoked a cigarette in the last year, and one third more the percentage of weekly smokers have smoked a cigarette in the last month. These additional students represent a substantial number of those at risk for regular adolescent and adult smoking, and programming needs to be sensitive to their orientation toward tobacco use. Conceivably, then, cessation or cessation support information would be relevant for approximately 45% of a high school class.

Classroom-based cessation programming offers three advantages compared to school-based cessation clinics or self-help programming (e.g., Burton, Sussman, Dent, et al., 1989). First, all students at high levels of tobacco use who are not absent from class are exposed to some cessation program information. Far fewer regular users are likely to be motivated enough to attend a clinic or read self-help material. On the other hand, fewer than 20% of regular adolescent or young adult tobacco users report no interest in quitting (Burton et al., 1994; Burton, Sussman, Dent, et al., 1989; Pallonen et al., 1990). A classroom cessation program may provide a major means of imparting the skills to enable many regular users to enter an action phase in the tobacco use cessation process. They might quit or at least learn some of the tools to quit after being exposed to this material. Second, potential future regular users also would be provided with cessation information in a way that provided a preventive function. Third, nonusers in the classroom are exposed to material on how to serve as support persons. Thus a better social environment for quitting might be created.

To our knowledge, the only published classroom-based cessation study was a 3-day smoking cessation program provided to 20 tenth-grade classes at four northern California high schools (Pallonen, 1987; Perry et al., 1983). A curriculum emphasizing social consequences was compared to a health consequences curriculum. Overall, 23% of the 82 weekly smokers in the sample quit at immediate posttest, and no difference in quit rate was found across the two conditions. More recent data indicate that both social influences and addiction-related material are relevant to adolescent cessation (Burton et al., 1994; Pallonen, 1987; Sussman et al., 1991). Thus a social influences approach along with material on addiction and quitting techniques would be most appropriate in the high school context.

Integrating Prevention and Cessation

The drawback of a cessation orientation would be if it were to make permissible tobacco experimentation for some students (e.g., those who believe they don't have to quit yet because cessation is not yet relevant to them; Pentz, Brannon, et al., 1989). Integrating prevention with cessation information would help minimize that potential difficulty. Prevention material could be used to suggest cessation as a last resort rather than as an attractive option. Such an integration would also maintain the relevance of programming for those whom cessation programming alone is not relevant (e.g., many nonusers or triers).

Several tobacco use education activities have been implemented across adult and adolescent prevention and cessation contexts (Burton, Sussman, Dent, et al., 1989; Burton et al., 1994). For example, learning assertiveness, dealing with direct social pressure to use tobacco, becoming aware of and counteracting subtle advertising and peer modeling influences, and making a commitment to not use tobacco are components of both types of programming. It also is the case that some knowledge and skill domains generally taught only in cessation programming are applicable not only to regular tobacco users and their support persons but also to anyone who is at risk for future tobacco addiction. For example, one component of cessation programming typically emphasizes "cues" or "triggers" for relapse, based on the well-established link between situational cues and addiction processes (e.g., Marlatt & Gordon, 1985). In adolescence, relapse cues (e.g., presence of others who smoke) are likely to pervade certain social settings, such as high-school-age parties (e.g., Sussman, Dent, Raynor, et al., 1988). Programming is needed to link acquired knowledge and skills to these potential "high-risk" situations so that program contents can become accessible enough from memory to effectively counteract pressures to use fostered by these settings. This is consistent with memory accessibility models of health behavior (Stacy, Dent, et al., 1990; Stacy, MacKinnon, & Pentz, 1993). Establishing links between high-risk settings and program information could help counteract any tobacco experimentation (i.e., trial use or relapse prevention), and recently has been incorporated to some extent in prevention efforts (Sussman, 1989; Wills, 1986). Thus cessation-oriented components can be integrated with prevention into a more comprehensive approach. To maximize the chances of success of such a program, curriculum development testing is needed to develop and integrate prevention and cessation activities.

NEED FOR RESEARCH WITH HIGH-RISK POPULATIONS: THE EXAMPLE OF CONTINUATION HIGH SCHOOLS

A major issue when discussing the applicability of adolescent tobacco use or drug abuse prevention programming to higher risk settings is that "high risk" is a concept of varying meaning (Sussman, Simon, & Stacy, 1994). This term could refer to disadvantaged socioeconomic groups (within which drug use or distribution traditionally has been more prevalent), risk takers or those who identify with high-risk groups (Fishkin et al., 1993; Sussman et al., 1990; Sussman, Dent, Simon, et al., 1993), confirmed adolescent drug users or abusers; those who report lower perceived risk of negative consequences; those who are targets of drug promotions (e.g., of cigarettes and alcohol); and so on (e.g., Johnson et al., 1990). One widely shared perspective of high risk, particularly easy to conceptualize and operationalize in terms of social influence theory, is defined as "the percentage of users within a social environment" (Johnson et al., 1990; Sussman, Dent, Simon, et al., in press; Sussman, Stacy, et al., in press). The greater the number of users within a large (school, community) or small (e.g., peer group) social environment, the more at risk are its members. When schools are made the unit of study, schools differing in percentage of users at baseline reflect different levels of risk.

Continuation versus comprehensive (regular) high schools form a natural demarcation of youth who are at relatively high or low risk for substance use in California (Sussman, Dent, Simon, et al., in press; Sussman, Stacy, et al., in press). Before reaching high school in California, youth remain at the same elementary or junior high school. When reaching high school age, those youth who are unable to remain in the comprehensive school system for emotional, behavioral, or other functional reasons, including substance use, are transferred to a continuation school. Overall, use of tobacco in the past 30 days among regular high school students (averaged across grades) is approximately 32% nationally, and daily use is a approximately 15% (Johnston, O'Malley, & Bachman, 1993). Among continuation high school youth, use in the past 30 days is about 47% and 38% report daily use. Clearly, a much higher prevalence of tobacco use is evident at continuation high schools (Sussman, Dent, Simon, et al., in press; Sussman, Stacy, et al., in press).

Continuation high schools were established in 1919 pursuant to the California Educational Code (Section 48400), which requires continued (part-time) education for all California youth until they reach 18 years of age. Students who are experiencing life difficulties when beginning high school may choose to transfer to a continuation school, where hours are more flexible and the teacher to student ratio is twice as high as comprehensive schools (i.e., 1:15 versus 1:30). Every school district that has an enrollment of over 100 students in 12th grade must have a continuation school program; there are approximately 450 continuation high schools in the state of California.

An implicit goal of a continuation school is to channel students back into mainstream society. Effective substance abuse prevention for many of these students is imperative for them to achieve the goal of being mainstreamed. Unfortunately, most prevention programming has not been adapted or applied to such students (Sussman, Dent, Simon, et al., in press; Sussman, Stacy, et al., in press). Tobacco and drug abuse prevention programming is sorely needed because individuals at these schools may be at a critical juncture for either returning to the mainstream or transitioning to more problematic behaviors, including increased tobacco and other drug use leading to addiction/drug abuse. Thus, regarding need for tobacco and drug abuse prevention programming, students from continuation high schools represent an underserved as well as a high-risk population. Project Towards No Drug Abuse (Project TND) is a 5-year study funded by the National Institute on Drug Abuse to prevent drug abuse among continuation high school youth at 21 schools in southern California (investigators include Drs. Sussman, Stacy, Dent, and Johnson). This project will test the effects on school-level tobacco and other drug use between a classroom-only novel curriculum condition (involving social influence and other components; e.g., intrapersonal, chemical dependency oriented), a classroom-plus-school-as-community condition (where a student group, the Associated Student Body, extends out to the community), and a "standard care" control condition in a three-group randomized design. Many of the principles or lessons presented in this book are being applied to this recently funded project. This project will help extend curriculum development research from the testing of a curriculum for youth in the classroom to detailed assessment of the development of (a) a classroom curriculum for "high-risk" high school youth, (b) a school-as-community program, and (c) individualized instruction components that fall outside of typical classroom instruction.

"Vocational" and other "alternative" schools, as they are referred to elsewhere in the United States, are analogous to continuation high schools. They also show much higher prevalences of tobacco use than in regular high schools (e.g., Corcoran & Allegrante, 1989). In order to affect youth in these settings, programs need to (a) make students aware of the wider community that disapproves of tobacco and other drug use by bringing corrective information into the classroom, (b) make nonusers in these settings attractive role models for other youths, (c) expose youths to settings in which tobacco and other drug use is discouraged and to which they aspire (e.g., job settings), and (d) teach these youth skills to help them bridge to lower risk settings (e.g., alternative means of coping aside from tobacco use). Of course, one can't rule out integration of cessation with prevention material or use of cessation clinics in these settings because there is a higher prevalence of regular tobacco users. One recent study, which provided tobacco use cessation clinic programming for 60 youth at one continuation high school in southern California, was able to maintain clinic attendance of such youth over six sessions, though cessation of tobacco use was only 5% at a 6-week follow-up (Cinnamin, 1993). More research is needed to maximize the quality of cessation as well as prevention programming in higher risk settings.

NEED FOR THE STUDY OF PREVENTION AMONG ETHNIC MINORITIES: AFRICAN AMERICANS AS AN EXAMPLE

At least one study suggests that effects on disadvantaged ethnic groups may be favored in current comprehensive social influences tobacco and drug prevention programming (Graham, Johnson, Hansen, Flay, & Gee, 1990). On the other hand, African American adults in particular still show the highest rate of smoking of any ethnic group and are at highest risk for health consequences of smoking (Lopes, Sussman, Galaif, & Crippens, in press; Orleans, Stecher, Schoenbach, Salmon, & Blackmon, 1989), although relatively few African American adolescents have been found to smoke cigarettes in the past 30 days (5%), compared to white (15%) and Latino (10%) adolescents (U.S. DHHS, 1994, p. 61). Thus a great deal of current research is focused on developing culturally sensitive programming tailored to maximize impact on ethnic minorities, which acknowledges that African American adolescents begin to smoke at a slightly older age (1 to 2 years older) than young people from other ethnic groups (e.g., Parker & Sussman, 1994).

Cultural sensitivity refers to an awareness of and accommodation to the lifestyle of an identifiable group of people (e.g., Amuleru-Marshall, 1991). In certain subpopulations in this country, clear cultural distinctions exist that include use of a different language and adoption of cultural traditions obviously related to past residence in a country other than the United States. With African Americans, on the other hand, dialects of English are spoken, and centuries divide the African American from the traditions of a different country. In this country, African culture was drastically modified through necessary adjustments to a dominant, perhaps cruel, Anglo culture. Hence what is culturally unique among African Americans is more subtle (e.g., Amuleru-Marshall, 1991; Hilliard, 1976). To date, we lack a complete, empirically determined understanding of the unique characteristics of the lifestyle of African Americans. Certain distinctions have been noted regarding the black American life situation, particularly of those who have the lowest socioeconomic status, including:

1. Approximately 38% of black households are headed by a single female parent. Young black females are relatively more likely than whites or other racial or ethnic groups to rear children without the father's continuing presence in the home. Although young African American women may gain a sense of purpose by becoming pregnant, they may do so with the realization that they probably will raise the child virtually without the father (Anderson, 1991).

2. Young African Americans are at greater risk than other groups for low academic attainment, poor job skills, and underemployment or unemployment. Decreases in federal funding for a range of social service programs have resulted in little governmental support for them. For these reasons, the young African American remains mired in low socioeconomic status. The experience of child rearing in such circumstances is probably particularly difficult for the young mother (Anderson & McNeilly, 1991).

3. Hypersegregation is prevalent among African Americans (i.e., more poor blacks live next to poor blacks than poor whites live next to poor whites). Thus relatively fewer role models for upward mobility are present within a poor African American community, and greater psychological distress is reported (Anderson, 1991; Anderson & McNeilly, 1991).

4. Perhaps more than members of the dominant cultural group in the United States, African Americans may look to certain institutions to provide both tangible support and a more intangible sense of belonging. Two of these most readily identified institutions are the black church and the extended family (Anderson, 1991; Hilliard, 1976).

More is known about specific patterns of cigarette use among blacks than about components of the African American culture that predispose for or facilitate tobacco use among this group. Blacks and whites are similar in some regards—many of the perceived reasons for one's smoking and reasons to quit smoking are the same among African Americans and European Americans, for example (Lopes et al., in press; Parker et al., 1994)—but distinct differences do exist:

1. Although African Americans are not more likely to smoke than members of other groups, adult blacks are significantly less likely than whites to quit smoking. Also, the smoking rate among black women is declining more slowly than the rate for men or women in any other ethnic group (Orleans et al., 1989; Rogers & Crank, 1988).

2. Blacks are likely to show a unique low-rate/high-nicotine menthol-smoking pattern (Orleans et al., 1989).

3. Blacks show a relatively greater percentage of dependent smoking (e.g., smoking within 30 minutes of waking in the morning) (e.g., Lopes et al., in press).

4. Although most reasons for smoking are the same for blacks and whites, one relatively unique reason for beginning smoking among blacks may be as a means of sensation seeking or dealing with feelings of anger. Also, peer influences may be more relevant for the initiation of smoking among whites, and parental influences may be more relevant to blacks (Koepke, Flay, & Johnson, 1990; Parker & Sussman, 1994), although social influence prevention programs are at least as effective for blacks as for whites (Botvin et al., 1989; DeMoor, Elder, Young, Wildey, & Molgaard. 1989; Graham et al., 1990; Headen, Bauman, Deane, & Koch, 1991; Parker et al., 1994; Sussman et al., 1987). (This same research literature indicates that family influences and anger also are relatively important etiological predictors among Latinos; likewise, social influences prevention programming is effective among Latinos.)

5. A culturally unique reason for quitting smoking among blacks appears to be the perception that the church with which one affiliates holds negative attitudes toward smoking (Lopes et al., in press; Orleans et al., 1989).

6. Because they are related to moving out of poverty, use of empowerment-related strategies probably are relevant to help African Americans to not begin or to quit smoking (e.g., emphasis on the family, the church, upward mobility, ethnic group pride, counteracting of the "beauty" of billboards advertising smoking in poor areas (e.g., Amuleru-Marshall, 1991).

7. Young black females prefer media role models who are African Americans living in life situations similar to their own (Lopes et al., in press).

Still, more information is needed to tap culturally unique dimensions relevant for inclusion in prevention programming targeted to this community. For example, reasons for the relative preference of menthol cigarettes among blacks are not clear. Some researchers have conjectured that menthol may permit deeper inhalation of tobacco smoke, permitting more nicotine intake per cigarette. Thus menthol cigarette smoking may represent a cost-effective nicotine regulation mechanism. Yet other social reasons are possible (e.g., ethnic identity, to demonstrate a difference from whites).

Also, young African Americans have concerns relevant to their age-specific experiences (e.g., greater number of black role models on TV, interest in rap music, crack as a drug of choice). Pregnant young females have unique concerns, including family perceptions of their pregnancy status and economic needs. Means of tailoring current programming to African Americans would be helpful. Finally, over the last 15 years, African American adolescents have reported a sharp decrease in prevalence of regular cigarette smoking, that is, in the last 30 days, whereas this decrease is not evident in whites (U.S. DHHS, 1994). More research is needed to examine why this is the case, as well as to examine whether (and if so, why) African American adolescents are more likely to show a steeper increase relative to whites in young adulthood (i.e., 18-24 years).

NEED FOR NOVEL INTERVENTION CONTEXTS

There are various community alternatives to classroom-based or school-based clinic programming. Smoking prevention programming at 4-H or Boys and Girls Clubs, taxation or other means of raising the price of tobacco products, enforcement of sales regulations at convenience stores, prevention messages aired on television or provided in the newspapers, minimal interventions provided by pediatricians or dentists in clinic settings, and parental-involvement-oriented programming all provide supplementary or alternative modalities. One novel alternative option to providing prevention or cessation information to youth of high school age is to bypass a school intervention entirely, such as by providing a *home telephone-based intervention,* as has been accomplished successfully by Project SHOUT (John Elder, personal communication; Elder et al., 1993). In this type of intervention, prevention agents phone adolescents at home. This approach is complementary to a school-based approach, and may be most relevant to use when students leave high school. Several potential problems remain with this alternative prevention method. Institutionalizing such an approach may be difficult; it may not be clear which institutions would be engaged in such an endeavor. Second, all students may not be able to be reached through phone calls. Third, biochemical validation of self-reports may be more difficult to accomplish than in a face-to-face approach. Finally, such an approach with present affordable technology may not able to provide certain benefits of face-to-face teaching (e.g., certain process elements of teaching may be lost, visual aspects of social skill development probably cannot be taught to criteria). This approach holds much promise in future public health efforts, but the above-mentioned difficulties need to be controlled for through future research.

NEED FOR PARTICIPATION IN PROGRAMMING BY SCHOOL PERSONNEL

As Role Models

Staff can model healthy behavior for their students. As instructors and adult role models, school personnel are the major institutional providers of health information to school-age children. Compared to others, healthy (e.g., nonsmoking) school staff are likely to be absent from school less often, project better morale, have more energy to teach or engage in other school duties, and be more supportive of health education programming for students, and they are more likely to model healthy behavior for the many students with whom they are in contact with during the day (Blair, Tritsch, & Kutsch, 1987; Chen & Winder, 1985). Alternatively, staff smoking could influence students to smoke due to modeling effects or acceptance of staff smoking at any location on the school grounds.

The school context is an especially important one in which to introduce a no-smoking policy for school personnel because such a policy could have two effects: (a) to help these adults reduce or quit tobacco use and, in turn, achieve a more healthy lifestyle; and (b) to help reduce tobacco use among the student population. Prevalence of smoking among Project TNT school personnel was presented in Chapter 6.

Evans et al. (1979) were among the first to suggest that school personnel model smoking behavior for their students. Indeed, the school context is one where many youth are exposed to adult authority who are tobacco users. Data within and outside of our research group indicate that there is a positive association between student and school staff tobacco use (e.g., Bewley, Johnson, & Banks, 1979; Charlin et al., 1990; McNeill et al., 1988; Murray, Kiryluk, & Swan, 1984; Pentz et al., 1990). Although most staff smoking in southern California public schools is limited to designated staff lounges (Barovich et al., 1988), many staff do not follow those rules, still show evidence of tobacco use on their person (e.g., cigarette packs in their pockets or tobacco odor on their clothes), and throw cigarette butts about the school campus (Charlin et al., 1990). Furthermore, the fact that a smoking area is provided (even informally) may legitimize use to students (Barovich et al., 1988; Sussman, 1989). School personnel report concern about exposing students to their smoking (Nutbeam, 1987) and have been motivated to participate and become healthier through involvement in health promotion programming at school (e.g., Blair et al., 1984). A no-smoking policy on the school grounds could facilitate smoking cessation among personnel and affect students' attitudes and behavior regarding smoking. Unfortunately, a majority of school personnel who are smokers do not see themselves as partly responsible for student smoking, and they desire to be able to continue to smoke in staff lounges (Galaif, Sussman, & Bundek, 1994).

As Teachers of Tobacco Use Prevention

Teacher training permits school health teachers to continue to deliver prevention curricula to students. Likewise, staff-run clinics provide a means to permit a cessation program to continue to be implemented at the school. School nurses or physical education teachers might be those best suited to provide cessation clinics to students. Thus certain teachers are the ones that keep or don't keep an effective tobacco use prevention or cessation program implemented in the schools. The support of the school principal also can help these teachers keep these types of programs going (Rohrbach et al., 1993).

Some people have assumed, on the other hand, that use of same-aged peers or older peers as providers of prevention or cessation programming would be superior to use of adults (discussed in Flay, 1985; Johnson, 1981). The trade-off really is between relative importance of student identification with another student versus student perceptions of expertise, the latter of which are more likely to be attributed to adults. The "bottom line" of our work and the work of others is that a good teacher—student or adult—is what's important. However, there must be sufficient training and incentives to enable teachers to provide maximum programming in appropriate classes (as discussed later in this chapter). Use of a student as an instructor, though relatively cost-effective in terms of teaching costs, may require more training than use of seasoned adult teachers, and students are only likely to be able to teach a prevention course a few times (before they graduate). School teachers are our "best bet" for continuing to deliver good prevention programs at schools.

NEED FOR NEW THEORETICAL ORIENTATIONS: THE EXAMPLE OF MEMORY AND INFORMATION-PROCESSING APPROACHES TO TOBACCO USE ETIOLOGY AND PREVENTION

It should be emphasized that the social psychological foundations of Project TNT, as well as all other large tobacco use prevention efforts, have centered on "dimensional" theories and methods (Devine & Ostrom, 1988; Ostrom, 1990). Dimensional approaches assume that social and cognitive processes can be studied by variations along dimensions measured on scales such as self-efficacy, outcome expectancies for social approval, and other constructs. Dimensional approaches are in line with traditional social influence theories from the 1950s and 1960s, as well as some refinements based on social learning theory. These approaches are in contrast to the largest movement in social psychology in the 1980s and 1990s—information-processing approaches to social cognition. As Devine and Ostrom pointed out, social psychology went through what some individuals have called a paradigm shift in the late 1970s, away from dimensional theories and toward information-processing approaches. Although the information-processing approach in social psychology may actually represent something less than a paradigm shift in that dimensional approaches are still commonly used, information-processing approaches are certainly the predominant focus in social psychology today. We do not argue that recent and current fashion necessarily implies superiority, but there are many reasons to argue for the usefulness of an information-processing approach.

Information-processing approaches assume there are many cognitive processes involved in behavior change, and that most of these processes are not necessarily measurable by self-reports on typical (dimensional) questionnaire measures of social or drug use variables. Some of the fundamental variables in information-processing approaches include attentional focus, context, compatibility in cognitive processing, memory encoding, elaboration, and storage, memory association, and memory retrieval or activation. From this perspective, most questionnaire responses are not likely to reflect long-term memory or any long-term predisposition, but may instead reflect a host of judgment processes inherent in answering a questionnaire (Feldman & Lynch, 1988; Wyer & Srull, 1989). For example, many questionnaire responses are strongly influenced by one's working memory for previous answers to the questionnaire, the questionnaire administration context, and other factors.

In Project TNT, we at least began to investigate a few information-processing variables, using the memory framework espoused by Stacy and his colleagues (e.g., Stacy, 1994; Stacy, Dent, et al., 1990; Stacy, Galaif, Sussman, & Dent, 1994; Stacy, Leigh, & Weingardt, in press). For example, in Stacy, Dent, et al. (1990), we found that a simple manipulation of the accessibility from memory of subject thoughts about certain drug use outcomes (e.g., good or bad outcomes) strongly influenced whether a questionnaire variable (expectancy about positive outcomes) was or was not predictive of tobacco use intentions. The effect was dramatic because the prediction of intention was strong when positive outcomes were made accessible from memory and totally absent otherwise. This study demonstrated the extremely dynamic nature of questionnaire responses and of constructs that in dimensional approaches are assumed to be fairly stable or measurable without acknowledgment of memory processes.

More recently, we have found support for the use of a wide variety of implicit memory tests in drug use. These tests assess memory associations between different types of drugs and perceived outcomes involved in drug use (Stacy et al., in press), as well as memory associations among features of drug use situations (Stacy, 1994). These types of tests, which are compatible with the information-processing perspective, can be used to assess baseline memory associations that are involved in drug use, as well as changes in memory associations as a result of a prevention program. With respect to alcohol use, implicit memory for alcohol effects appears to be involved in the cognitive mediation of alcohol abuse. Subsequent research may find that this is also true for tobacco and other drug use. The National Institute on Drug Abuse recently acknowledged that the memory mediators of drug use may be among the most fundamental determinants of drug craving (Swan, 1993).

Information-processing perspectives can also be used to reinterpret many findings in prevention research. Although the content of prevention activities undoubtedly is important, the specific cognitive processes engaged in these activities are just as important. Unfortunately, different prevention curricula usually confound likely differences in cognitive processing and content. For example, some curricula may inadvertently encourage processing that is compatible with the types of processing that actually occur during high-risk social situations, in which the student may be encouraged (implicitly or explicitly) to use tobacco. Another program may not encourage such compatibility. One program may encourage elaborative processing and be implemented in a way that guarantees that each student engages in elaborative processing, whereas another program may not. One should consider the possibility that elaborative processing may be a reason for the success of our physical consequences curricula, for example, whereas typical physical consequence curricula may not have engaged the students in this type of processing. The main point here is to suggest that information-processing variables should be a focus of prevention research because (a) they are a likely confound with the content of many programs, (b) they have shown strong influences on cognitive responses and behavior in numerous studies in basic research and other areas of applied research (e.g., marketing, advertising), and (c) they are a primary focus of modern social and cognitive psychology. On the basis of these considerations, there is a tremendous amount of room for improvement in the development of prevention campaigns and their evaluation in tobacco and drug use. Although dimensional approaches have shown enough success to be implemented, effects have sometimes been weak, and results are often mixed or likely to quickly dissipate. Information-processing perspectives, with their focus on the dynamic and highly conditional nature of human cognition and memory, could very well bring new life into prevention efforts. Consequently these efforts may become better competitors against the promoters of tobacco use, whose advertising agencies have used information-processing approaches for a number of years.

ARE WE REALLY READY
FOR TECHNOLOGY TRANSFER?

Diffusion is defined as the spread of new knowledge, usually referred to as an innovation, to a defined population over time through specific channels. *Innovations* are ideas, practices, or objects that are perceived as new by units of adoption (Rogers, 1983). The diffusion of innovative school-based programs is characterized as a four-stage process (Parcel et al., 1989; Rogers, 1983; Best, Thomson, Santi, Smith, & Brown, 1988). The first stage is dissemination, in which school districts are made aware of new, successful programs and are encouraged to adopt them. The second stage is adoption, in which districts make a commitment to initiate a program. The third stage, implementation, occurs when teachers or other appropriate personnel deliver the program. The final stage is maintenance, in which school administrators and teachers are encouraged to continue use of the program.

The first stage, dissemination, generally stems from a consensus on what constitutes effective programming. Glynn (1989) outlines the consensus-derived essential features of adolescent smoking prevention programs, including providing at least seven lessons, teaching awareness of social influences, and teaching refusal assertion skills. Although much is agreed on, Johnson (1981) cautions against assuming we have all the answers (e.g., different content may be relevant for different youth, need for peer leaders is questionable). McCaul & Glasgow (1985) further challenge what is known about the research area in terms of effects mediation. Indeed, MacKinnon et al. (1991) found that peer approval, positive outcome expectancies for drug effects, and prevalence estimates, rather than refusal assertion skills instruction, mediated effects obtained in the Midwestern Prevention Project. Previously, we described other confounds in social influence programs. Even though previous multicomponent programs have achieved successful preventive outcomes, the effectiveness of many individual program components either has not been tested or has not been found to mediate prevention program successes (Johnson, 1981; McCaul & Glasgow, 1985). These findings are not surprising, considering the tendency for formative evaluation to be less carefully done than summative evaluation (Evans et al., 1989). There is some uncertainty about why these programs work because mediators of change have not been carefully tested throughout the curriculum development process. Clearly, more research is needed to understand the processes of behavior change.

Even after a program is deemed successful, it still may not become owned by a community (adopted). Project TNT has been adopted by our school districts, however, simply because we have had ongoing contact with them for 5 years and because we provided free teacher training for them (using the combined condition). Even if a program is adopted, it may not be implemented for long. A means of keeping a program implemented, and implemented intact, after the researchers leave the scene is of great importance to the future of prevention research. For example, Rohrbach et al. (1993) found that implementation of a drug abuse prevention program by trained junior high school teachers, as a means of disseminating Project AAPT (Alcohol Abuse Prevention

Trials), is not particularly successful at present. Although about 80% of trained teachers implemented one or more lessons after training (n = 60 teachers), only 25% maintained implementation the next year. Implementers reported fewer years of teaching experience and more enthusiasm for delivery of the program. Encouragement by the school principal, not intensive teacher training, increased rates of implementation. As of yet, we are not sure of the extent to which Project TNT will continue to be implemented in our districts.

Are we ever ready for diffusion of tobacco use prevention and cessation school-based programming? Maybe, but perhaps only if we are prepared to recycle through the steps of program development. We believe that as researchers begin to engage in diffusion of existing curricula, there is increasing need for curricula refinement studies to adapt curricula to new circumstances. The four-step model presented in Chapter 7 should be useful for researchers and practitioners in their efforts to develop efficacious school-based prevention studies in new contexts (Sussman, 1991). An abridged sequence of steps could be used. A needs assessment should disclose any relevant antecedent or perceived consequence variables of the risk behavior in that new context. Focus groups or theme studies should be used to provide discussion regarding what aspects of a curriculum need modification to work with a particular subpopulation. Component studies should allow for tests of immediate effects of modified lessons. Likewise, some piloting would help to "smooth out the rough edges" of adaptations and help us to assess whether the curriculum has or has not lost impact on immediate outcomes compared to its original version. Finally, there is a need to engage in technology transfer research, with an emphasis on maximizing implementation and maintenance of a program over the next several years following the termination of a research program.

Of course, even if programs do not work in and of themselves, they may establish a context for social change. In the context of other legislative, preventive, and cessation efforts, gradual widespread impact on tobacco use might occur. This impact might not be detectable for several years. Thus even though it is better to provide a complete and effective school-based tobacco use prevention or cessation program, one may argue that provision of almost *any* programming is better than none. On the other hand, it is possible for programs to exert *negative* effects, although most such programs are not reported in the research literature (e.g., Hansen, Johnson, et al., 1988). Even if a program might exert delayed positive effects, or contribute to an anti-tobacco-use social milieu, good research dictates that the process of such effects be *specified* to produce better future programs. Research should continue searching for the set of processes most responsible for behavior change.

CONCLUSIONS

In this book we have attempted to provide myriad details about school-based tobacco use prevention and cessation research and programming, ideas that could be used by researchers, practitioners, policy makers, and students. Our description of this type of research and programming was built around our grant funded by the National Cancer Institute for Project TNT. We continue our effort in continuation high schools, Project TND (Towards No Drug Abuse), on a grant funded by the National Institute on Drug Abuse.

We hope we leave the reader with a taste of our shared orientation to this research area. It all starts out with a theoretical framework. Then we try to link all developmental work through empirical studies. We try to engage in field experimental evaluations of our work and control for alternative interpretations of our condition manipulations. We carefully evaluate our outcomes, and we maintain a healthy skepticism regarding diffusion of programming though continued research. In this book, we focused our efforts on the school context, not on other contexts, though these other settings also are very important to investigate. We believe there is still much more to learn about when engaging in health research in schools. We hope that we provide material that can assist the reader to prepare his or her own service delivery, evaluation, or research study, and we look forward to maximizing the effectiveness of tobacco use prevention and cessation programming on youth (of all ages).

Project Towards No Tobacco Use
Prevention Curricula Contents

	Combined Condition	Informational Social Influence Condition	Normative Social Influence Condition	Physical Consequences Condition
Lesson 1	Active Listening	Active Listening	Active Listening	Active Listening
Lesson 2	Consequences Course	Tobacco Prevalence	Ingratiation	Consequences Course
Lesson 3	Self-Esteem	Values	Cognitive Restructuring	Addiction
Lesson 4	Ingratiation/ Cognitive Restructuring	Advertising Images	Refusal Learning	Diseases
Lesson 5	Effective Communication	Self-Esteem	Avoidance	Cost of Addiction
Lesson 6	Refusal Learning	Effective Communication	Refusal Practice	Horrific Images
Lesson 7	Refusal Practice	Starting/ Maintaining Conversations	Refusal Practice	Sean Marsee Memorial
Lesson 8	Advertising Images	Social Problem Solving	Escape and Stress Management	Risk of Consequences
Lesson 9	Social Activism	Social Image Activism	Social Activism	Consequences Advocacy
Lesson 10	Public Commitment	Public Commitment	Public Commitment	Public Commitment

SOURCE: Adapted from Sussman, Dent, Stacy, Hodgson, et al., 1993.

Project TNT Combined Curriculum Lessons Preview

Lesson/Title	Description
1 Active Listening	Students are introduced to Project TNT and discuss the importance of being active listeners.
2 The Course of Tobacco Use and Consequences	Students learn about the course of tobacco addition and disease through role playing and will identify the consequences associated with tobacco use.
3 Self-Esteem	Students practice techniques to improve their self-esteem by learning to acknowledge their own positive characteristics.
4 Ingratiation and Cognitive Restructuring	Students are introduced to peer pressure and discuss how they can deal with peer pressure and still be liked by their friends. In addition, students learn about "thought-changing" processes in order to realize that peer pressure situations are not always as threatening as they initially appear.
5 Effective Communication	Students are introduced to the importance of effective communication. They practice good listening skills and initiating conversations, and learn how to effectively use open-ended questions.
6 Refusal Learning	Students learn the importance of being assertive and are introduced to various ways of saying "no."
7 Refusal Practice	Students view a film depicting the different ways to say no and then practice these methods.
8 Advertising Images	Students discuss the ways in which the media portray tobacco "social images" that influence individuals to use tobacco. A film discussing tobacco advertising images is viewed.

continued

Appendix B Continued

9 Social Activism	Students discuss what it means to be a social activist and practice being one by writing letters advocating no tobacco use.
10 Public Commitment Using Videotaping	Each class makes a video using a news program format. The students summarize what they have learned in Project TNT. Each student answers a question and shares a commitment he or she has made regarding tobacco use.

APPENDIX C

Project TNT Informational Social Influence Curriculum Lessons Preview

Lesson/Title	Description
1 Active Listening	Students are introduced to Project TNT and discuss the importance of being active listeners.
2 Tobacco Prevalence	Students will compare the assumed prevalence of tobacco use with the actual use.
3 Values	Students will discuss ways to achieve "healthy" values and the images they desire without tobacco use.
4 Advertising Images	Students will discuss the ways in which the media portray tobacco "images" that influence individuals to use tobacco. A film discussing tobacco advertising will be viewed.
5 Self-Esteem	Students will practice techniques to improve their self-esteem by learning to acknowledge their own positive characteristics.
6 Effective Communication	Students will identify three major parts of communication and will practice role-play situations to enhance good communication and assertiveness.
7 Starting and Keeping Conversations Going	Students will practice how to develop open-ended questions in order to make communication easier.
8 Social Problem Solving	Students will identify four steps in information gathering and decision making.
9 Social Activism	Students will discuss what it means to be a social activist and will practice by writing letters advocating no tobacco use.

continued

Appendix C Continued

10 Public Commitment Using Videotaping	Each class makes a video using a news program format. The students summarize what they have learned in Project TNT. Each student will answer a question and share a commitment he or she has made regarding tobacco use.

Project TNT Normative Social Influence Curriculum Lessons Preview

Lesson/Title	Description
1 Active Listening	Students are introduced to Project TNT and discuss the importance of being active listeners.
2 Ingratiation	Students are introduced to direct and indirect peer pressure and discuss how they can deal with it effectively and still be liked and accepted.
3 Cognitive Restructuring	Students are introduced to a thought-changing process in order to realize that situations are not always as threatening as they initially appear.
4 Refusal Learning	Students learn the importance of being assertive and are introduced to the various ways to say "no."
5 Avoidance	Students are introduced to the "KAT" avoidance method, which uses a decision-making process.
6 Film and Refusal Practice	Students view a film depicting ways to say "no," and then practice using these methods through a role play.
7 Refusal Practice	Students practice ways to say "no" through role playing.
8 Escape, Peer Pressure, and Stress Management	Students practice escape methods and then are introduced to stress reduction techniques.
9 Social Activism	Students will discuss what it means to be a social activist and will practice by writing letters advocating no tobacco use.
10 Public Commitment Using Videotaping	Each class will make a video using a news program format. The students will summarize what they have learned in Project TNT. Each student will answer a question and share a commitment he or she has made regarding tobacco use.

Project TNT Physical Consequences Curriculum Lessons Preview

Lesson/Title	Description
1 Active Listening	Students are introduced to Project TNT and discuss the importance of being active listeners.
2 Introduction to Consequences	Students will identify consequences of using tobacco and learn decision-making skills.
3 Addiction	Students will learn about the course of addition through role-play demonstration and the discussion of withdrawal symptoms.
4 Diseases	Students will discuss the diseases associated with tobacco use and their symptoms.
5 Cost of Addiction	Students will calculate the cost of addiction and identify facts regarding tobacco by playing "prevention baseball."
6 Anagrams and Horrific Images	Students will practice imagery to identify with negative consequences of tobacco use.
7 Sean Marsee Memorial	Students will discuss the death of Sean Marsee from smokeless tobacco use. They will also begin preparation and practice of a presentation about tobacco use consequences.
8 Risk of Consequences and Class Presentation	Students will identify the risk of disease in relation to tobacco use. Students will also perform presentations showing the consequences of tobacco use.
9 Consequence Advocacy	Students will discuss what it means to be an advocate and will practice by writing letters advocating no tobacco use.

continued

| 10 | Public Commitment Using Videotaping | Each class will make a video using a news program format. The students will summarize what they have learned in Project TNT. Each student will answer a question and share a commitment he or she has made regarding tobacco use. |

Outline of Project TNT Psychosocial-Oriented Cessation Clinic

Session 1   Subjects complete preclinic questionnaire. Subjects then introduce themselves and engage in a "scavenger hunt" ice breaker exercise. The purpose of the group and ground rules are provided. Next, reasons for using tobacco are mentioned. Students are focused on reasons of pleasure and managing stress, how to not give in to those tobacco use functions, and how to find alternative means of obtaining pleasure and coping with stress. Subjects pick a quit day between now and the third session, choose a means of quitting, and make a commitment to quit. Subjects receive the adult group leader's business card, quarters for support group phone calling, and a psychosocial-oriented audiotape.

Session 2   Subjects are complimented on attendance. Subjects set quit day and write down statement of commitment to quit. Subjects then review some of the physiological effects of tobacco use. They see brief films— *The Simple Surgeon*, a summary clip about Chew and Sean Marsee, and *Feminine Mistake*—with open discussions between each clip. Discussions emphasize cancer, heart disease, other conditions made worse from tobacco use, synergistic effects, and the effects of passive smoking. A CO monitor demonstration then is accomplished, a subject volunteer is assigned to make reminder calls for next meeting, the leader passes out another business card and handout, and subjects are reminded of quit day.

Session 3   Subjects are complimented on attendance. Subjects discuss their experiences of trying to quit tobacco use over the past week, and renewed goals are obtained from those who did not completely quit. Subjects discuss withdrawal symptoms and dependency symptoms (e.g., depression). Substitute behaviors, stress management, healthy breathing, the "floating" relaxation exercise, and cognitive coping are taught as coping strategies. Subjects are taught to practice coping strategies, set short-term and long-term goals, and discuss coping over the next few weeks. The leader describes the 3-month review session, distributes consent forms, and business card if necessary, and reminds everyone to refer to the information in his or her folder. A subject volunteer is assigned to make reminder phone calls, a handout is passed out, and the next meeting is briefly described.

Session 4   Subjects are greeted and acknowledged individually. Enthusiasm is promoted before going into content of the session. Each subject is asked, "What does it feel like to be conquering this dependency?" After this, the floating exercise is used to relax and visualize attainment of quitting goal. Stress management is discussed, focusing on anger (i.e., what makes you angry? how do express it?). Expressing anger constructively is taught (by being assertive). Another stressor is feeling down. Participants are asked, "What helps you to feel better when you are down?" Taking action against depression is taught as including identifying people "who make you feel good about yourself," "learning to be a good friend to yourself," and "being active." The leader asks, "who has questions about how to handle situations in the next few weeks," selects new phone volunteer, congratulates everyone's efforts and achievements, and reminds subjects to refer to their personal commitment statement, call each other for help, and come to next session.

Session 5   Subjects are greeted and acknowledged. Sharing is promoted to warm up and then subjects are asked, "Who can really *feel* that they are tobacco-free already?" Maintenance is discussed in terms of future plans and weight management. Assertively asking for good support and "Changing Versus Telling Us" are discussed. Emphasis is on striving hard to change what you can but letting go of things you cannot change. To accomplish this it helps to be tough but forgiving of yourself, using physical exercise like brisk walking, and using the floating exercise. Subjects are given another copy of audiocassette to give to a friend, complete a questionnaire, and are reminded about importance of attending a 3-month review session. A new phone volunteer is selected, and the leader encourages subjects to call each other for help, problems, and/or questions.

Outline of Project TNT
Addiction-Oriented Cessation Clinic

Session 1   Subjects are given preclinic questionnaire to complete. Subjects then
             introduce themselves and engage in a "scavenger hunt" ice breaker
             exercise. The purpose of the group and ground rules are mentioned.
             Students are focused on nicotine addiction: the definition, how we
             know it's addictive, comparisons to other drugs, how smokeless
             tobacco is more quickly addicting than cigarettes. The leader gives
             his or her personal experience with tobacco and other addictions.
             Subjects are asked how many think they are addicted to nicotine and
             discuss what it takes to become addicted. The experience of breaking
             an addiction is discussed as are means of withdrawal (drug
             withdrawal and body getting normal). Subjects pick a quit day
             between now and the third session, choose a means of quitting, and
             make a commitment to quit. Subjects receive the adult group leader's
             business card, quarters for support group phone calling, and an
             addiction-oriented audiotape.
Session 2   Subjects are complimented on attendance. Subjects set quit day and
             write down statement of commitment to quit. Subjects then review
             some of the physiological effects of tobacco use. They see brief films—
             The Simple Surgeon, a summary clip about Chew and Sean Marsee,
             and Feminine Mistake—with open discussions between each clip.
             Discussions emphasize cancer, heart disease, other conditions made
             worse from tobacco use, synergistic effects, and the effects of passive
             smoking. A CO monitor demonstration then is accomplished, a
             subject volunteer is assigned to make reminder calls for next meeting,
             the leader passes out another business card and handout, and
             subjects are reminded of quit day. This session is identical to the one
             in the psychosocial condition except that no psychosocial functions
             are discussed by the group leader.

Session 3   Subjects are complimented on attendance. Subjects discuss their experiences of trying to quit tobacco use over the past week, and renewed goals are obtained from those who did not completely quit. Nicotine withdrawal symptoms are discussed, how long they last, strategies to manage them, including physical exercise, and substitute behaviors. The floating exercise is introduced so subjects can relax and visualize their quit goal. Questions are elicited about how to handle next few weeks and a new phone volunteer is selected. The leader describes the 3-month review session, distributes consent forms and business card if necessary, and reminds everyone to refer to the information in his or her folder. A subject volunteer is assigned to make reminder phone calls, a handout is passed out, and next meeting is briefly described. This session is similar to the one in the psychosocial condition except that cognitive coping to counteract signals of psychosocial dependency for tobacco use is not included.

Session 4   Subjects are greeted and acknowledged individually. Enthusiasm is promoted before the content of the session is introduced. Each subject is asked, "What does it feel like to be conquering this dependency?" After this, the floating exercise is used so subjects can relax and visualize attainment of their quit goal. Withdrawal strategies from the past week are discussed. The first 3 months of cessation are discussed, strategies for dealing with maintaining cessation are discussed (e.g., coping with urges), and reasons for weight gain are given. The leader asks, "Who has questions about how to handle situations in the next few weeks," selects a new phone volunteer, congratulates everyone's efforts and achievements, and reminds subjects to refer to their personal commitment statement, call each other for help, and come to next session.

Session 5   Leader greets and acknowledges each individual and promotes sharing. The participants are asked, "Who can really *feel* that they are tobacco free already?" and a discussion is encouraged. The group talks about maintaining cessation—how it is enhanced by practical physical exercise like dancing, swimming, or walking, doing something different in daily routine, using the floating exercise, and reviewing personal commitment. Addiction as it applies to other drugs is discussed; what subjects have learned can be used in breaking other addictions but could be more difficult, and subjects can share the strategies they have learned with others. Subjects are given another copy of the audiocassette to give to a friend, complete a questionnaire, and are reminded about the importance of attending a 3-month review session. A new phone volunteer is selected, and the leader encourages subjects to call each other for help, problems, and/or questions.

APPENDIX H

Results of Selected Recent Smokeless Tobacco Prevention and Cessation Studies

A. Recent School-Based Programs Which Prevent Smokeless Tobacco Use

Name of Project	Target Group	Curricula	Number of Lessons	Teachers	Effects
Oregon Research Institute Study	7th and 9th graders	Comprehensive social influences, more normative social influence-oriented	7 lessons	Classroom teachers and peers	Effects on smokeless tobacco (males), not cigarettes, one year later; increase of .3 versus 4.7 chews per month (junior high school); decrease of 3.8 versus increase of 5.5 chews per month (high school); collapsed across genders and grade, increase of 13.2 versus 7.5 cigarettes per month (intervention versus control, not significant)
Project Towards No Tobacco Use (TNT)	7th graders	4 curricula: (a) physical consequences, (b) normative social influence (acceptability), (c) infor-	10 lessons, 2 booster lessons one year later	Health educators	Effects on both tobacco products in 8th and 9th grades: trial cigarettes (all program conditions, .07 versus .11 increase per year); weekly cigarettes

	7th graders	mational social influence (social images and prevalence), and (d) combined social influences and physical consequences; five conditions			(combined best, .02 versus .05 increase per year); trial smokeless tobacco (physical consequences best, .00 versus .03 increase per year, combined worked at 1-year only); weekly smokeless tobacco (physical consequences and combined best, –.005 decrease versus .005 increase per year)
Project SHOUT	7th graders	Comprehensive social influences	10 lessons in 7th grade, 8 lessons in 8th grade, 4 phone-call followups in 9th grade	Undergraduate college students	Effects on both tobacco products in 9th grade, .51 for smokeless tobacco, .69 for smoking, odds of past week tobacco use intervention versus control

261

B. Smokeless Tobacco Cessation Studies

Name of Researchers	Content	Number of Sessions	Subjects	Effects
Glover (1986)	Adapted the ACS's FreshStart program; clinics	4 sessions	41 18-to-22 year old adults, not voluntary	6-month abstinence of 2%
Eakin, Severson, & Glasgow (1989)	Coping skills training; clinics	3 small group sessions	25 14-to-18 year olds (5 poly-tobacco users)	6-month abstinence of 12%
DiLorenzo, Kern, & Pieper (1991)	Based on operant models, ACS-type programs; clinics	8 small group sessions	8 young adults	9-month abstinence of 75%
Zavela, Harrison, & Owens (1991)	Mint snuff, gum, lecture-only conditions; clinics	9 sessions	42 young adults	6-month abstinence of 29%, no difference among these conditions
Burton et al., (see U.S.D.H.H.S., 1994)	2 curricula, psychosocial and chemical dependency groups; clinics	6 small group sessions	60 14-to-18 year olds (12 poly-tobacco users)	3-month abstinence of 13% compared to 0% among wait-list controls, no significant difference across program conditions
Chakravorty (1992)	Mint snuff, gum, lecture-only conditions	2 small group sessions	83 14-to-18 year olds	Immediate posttest abstinence of 13%, no difference among these conditions
Stevens et al., (1992)	Dentist health care provider minimal intervention; exam, risks, advice, video and self-help	1-3 brief meetings	576 adults	12-month abstinence of 10%

References

Abrams, C., Selski, E., Craig, S., Barovich, M., & Sussman, S. (1989). *Project Towards No Tobacco Use (TNT): Tobacco use prevention guide, normative social influence curriculum*. Los Angeles: University of Southern California, Institute for Health Promotion and Disease Prevention Research.

Ajzen, I., & Fishbein, M. (1970). The prediction of behavior from attitudinal and normative variables. *Journal of Experimental Social Psychology, 6*, 466-487.

Ajzen, I., & Fishbein, M. (1980). *Understanding attitudes and predicting social behavior*. Englewood Cliffs, NJ: Prentice Hall.

Alexander, C. S., & Klassen, A. C. (1988). Drug use and illnesses among eighth grade students in rural schools. *Public Health Reports, 103*(4), 394-399.

Allen, V. L., & Wilder, D. A. (1980). Impact of group consensus and social support on stimulus meaning: Mediation and conformity by cognitive restructuring. *Journal of Personality and Social Psychology, 39*, 1116-1124.

Altman, D. G., Foster, V., Rasinick-Douss, L., & Tye, J. B. (1989). Reducing the illegal sale of cigarettes to minors. *Journal of the American Medical Association, 261*(1), 80-83.

Amuleru-Marshall, O. (1991). *Culturally-appropriate refinements in AIDS prevention among African-Americans*. Unpublished manuscript.

Anderson, C. L., & Creswell, W. H. (1976). *School health practice*. St. Louis: C. V. Mosby.

Anderson, N. (1991, March). *Keynote address*. Paper presented at the Society of Behavioral Medicine Twelfth Annual Scientific Sessions, Washington, DC.

Anderson, N. B., & McNeilly, M. (1991). Age, gender, and ethnicity as variables in psychophysiological assessment: Sociodemographics in context. *Psychological Assessment: A Journal of Consulting and Clinical Psychology, 3*, 376-384.

Ary, D. V., & Biglan, A. (1988). Longitudinal changes in adolescent cigarette smoking behavior: Onset and cessation. *Journal of Behavioral Medicine, 11*(4), 361-382.

Ary, D. V., Lichtenstein, E., Severson, H., Weissman, W., & Seeley, J. R. (1989). An in-depth analysis of male adolescent smokeless tobacco users: Interview with users and their fathers. *Journal of Behavioral Medicine, 12*, 449-467.

Atkins, N. P. (1978). Assessing community needs: Implications for curriculum and staff development in health education. *Journal of School Health, 48*(4), 220-224.

Bachman, J. G., O'Malley, P. M., & Johnston, L. D. (1984). Drug use among young adults: The impacts of role status and social environment. *Journal of Personality and Social Psychology, 47*, 629-645.

Bandura, A. (1977). *Social learning theory.* Englewood Cliffs, NJ: Prentice Hall.

Barcikowski, R. S. (1981). Statistical power with group means as the unit of analysis. *Journal of Educational Statistics, 6*, 267-285.

Baron, R. M., & Kenny, D. A. (1986). The moderator-mediator variable distinction in social psychological research: Conceptual, strategic, and statistical considerations. *Journal of Personality and Social Psychology, 51*(6), 1173-1182.

Barovich, M., Craig, S., Selski, E., Abrams, C., & Sussman, S. (1989). *Project Towards No Tobacco Use (TNT). Tobacco use prevention guide, informational social influences curriculum.* Los Angeles: University of Southern California, Institute for Health Promotion and Disease Prevention Research.

Barovich, M., Sussman, S., Dent, C. W., Burton, D., & Flay, B. R. (1991). Availability of tobacco products at stores located near public schools. *International Journal of the Addictions, 26*(8), 837-850.

Barovich, M., Sussman, S., Galaif, J., Dent, C. W., & Charlin, V. L. (1988). *School and store interview-to-observation studies. Phase 1: Assessment studies A and B, Project Towards No Tobacco Use (TNT)* (Technical Report #88-TNT-02). Los Angeles: University of Southern California, Institute for Health Promotion and Disease Prevention Research.

Basch, C. E. (1987). Focus group interview: An underutilized research technique for improving theory and practice in health education. *Health Education Quarterly, 14*, 411-448.

Basch, C. E., DeCicco, I. M., & Malfetti, J. L. (1989). A focus group study on decision processes of young drivers: Reasons that may support a decision to drink and drive. *Health Education Quarterly, 16*, 389-396.

Bauman, K. E., & Chenowith, R. L. (1984). The relationship between the consequences adolescents expect from smoking and their behavior: A factor analysis with panel data. *Journal of Applied Social Psychology, 14*, 28-41.

Bauman, K. E., & Dent, C. W. (1982). Influence of an objective measure on self-reports of behavior. *Journal of Applied Psychology, 67*, 623-628.

Bauman, K. E., Koch, G. G., Fisher, L. A., & Bryan, E. S. (1989). Use of smokeless tobacco by age, race, and gender in ten standard metropolitan statistical areas of the southeast United States. *National Cancer Institute Monographs, 8*, 35-37.

Baumrind, D. (1985). Family antecedents of adolescent drug use: A developmental perspective. In C. L. Jones & R. Battjes (Eds.), *Etiology of drug abuse: Implications for prevention* (NIDA Research Monograph 56) (pp. 13-44). Rockville, MD: National Institute on Drug Abuse.

Bellack, A. S., & Hersen, M. (1977). *Behavior modification.* Baltimore: Williams & Wilkins.

Belloc, N. B., & Breslow, L. (1972). Relationship of physical health status and health practices. *Preventive Medicine, 1*, 409-421.

Benfari, R. C., Ecker, E. D., Ockene, J., & McIntyre, K. (1982). Hyperstress and outcomes in a long-term smoking intervention program. *Psychometric Medicine, 44*, 227-235.

Berndt, T. J. (1979). Developmental changes in conformity to peers and parents. *Developmental Psychology, 15*(6), 608-616.

Best, J. A., Thomson, S. J., Santi, S. M., Smith, E. A., & Brown, K. S. (1988). Preventing cigarette smoking among school children. *Annual Review of Public Health, 9,* 161-201.

Bewley, B. R., Bland, J. M., & Harris, R. (1974). Factors associated with the starting of cigarette smoking by primary school children. *British Journal of Preventive and Social Medicine, 28,* 37-44.

Bewley, B. R., Johnson, M.R.D., & Banks, M. H. (1979). Teachers smoking. *British Journal of Preventive Medicine, 33,* 219-222.

Biglan, W., Severson, H., Ary, D., Faller, C., Gallison, C., Thompson, R., Glasgow, R., & Lichtenstein, E. (1987). Do smoking prevention programs really work? Attrition and the internal and external validity of an evaluation of a refusal skills training program. *Journal of Behavioral Medicine, 10,* 159-171.

Biglan, A., Weissman, W., & Severson, H. (1985). Coping with social influences to smoke. In S. Shiffman & T. A. Wills (Eds.), *Coping and substance use* (pp. 95-117). Orlando, FL: Academic Press.

Billings, A. G., & Moos, R. H. (1983). Social-environmental factors among light and heavy cigarette smokers: A controlled comparison with nonsmokers. *Addictive Behaviors, 8,* 381-391.

Blair, S. N., Collingwood, T. R., Reynolds, R., Smith, M., Hagan, D., & Sterling, C. L. (1984). Health promotion for educators: Impact on health behaviors, satisfaction, and general well-being. *American Journal of Public Health, 74*(2), 147-149.

Blair, S. N., Tritsch, L., & Kutsch, S. (1987). Worksite health promotion for school faculty and staff. *Journal of School Health, 57*(10), 469-473.

Bock, R. D. (1983). The discrete Bayesian. In H. Wainer (Ed.), *Modern advances in psychometric research.* New York: Lawrence Erlbaum.

Boring, E. G. (1957). *A history of experimental psychology* (chap. 1). Englewood Cliffs, NJ: Prentice Hall.

Borkovec, T. D., & Nau, S. D. (1972). Credibility of analogue therapy rationales. *Journal of Behavior Therapy and Experimental Psychiatry, 3,* 257-260.

Botvin, G. J. (1986). Substance abuse prevention research: Recent developments and future directions. *Journal of School Health, 56,* 369-374.

Botvin, G. J., Batson, H. W., Witts-Vitale, S., Bess, V., Baker, E., & Dusenbury, L. (1989). A psychosocial approach to smoking prevention for urban black youth. *Public Health Reports, 104*(6), 573-582.

Botvin, G. J., & Eng, A. (1979). *Life skills training: A comprehensive smoking prevention program.* New York: Smithfield.

Botvin, G. J., Renick, N. L., & Baker, E. (1983). The effects of scheduling format and booster sessions on a broad-spectrum psychosocial approach to smoking prevention. *Journal of Behavioral Medicine, 6,* 359-379.

Botvin, G. J., & Wills, T. A. (1985). Personal and social skills training: Cognitive-behavioral approaches to substance abuse prevention. In C. S. Bell & R. Battjes (Eds.), *Prevention research: Deterring drug abuse among children and adolescents* (NIDA Research Monograph 63). Rockville, MD: National Institute on Drug Abuse.

Boyd, G., & Associates (1987). Use of smokeless tobacco among children and adolescents in the United States. *Preventive Medicine, 16,* 402-421.

Boyd, G. M., & Glover, E. D. (1989). Smokeless tobacco use by youth in the U.S. *Journal of School Health, 59,* 189-194.

Brannon, B. R., Dent, C. W., Flay, B. R., Hansen, W. B., Johnson, C. A., Smith, G., & Sussman, S. (1989). The television, school, and family project: V. The impact of curriculum delivery format on program acceptance. *Preventive Medicine, 18,* 492-502.

Braverman, M. D., D'Onofrio, C. N., & Moskowitz, J. M. (1989). Marketing smokeless tobacco in California communities: Implications for health education. *National Cancer Institute Monographs, 8,* 79-85.

Brophy, J. (1986). Teacher influences on student achievement. *American Psychologist, 41,* 1069-1077.

Brown, B. B., & Lohr, M. J. (1987). Peer-group affiliation and adolescent self-esteem: An integration of ego-identity and symbolic-interaction theories. *Journal of Personality and Social Psychology, 52,* 47-55.

Brown, B. B., & Trujillo, C. M. (1985). *Adolescents' perceptions of peer group stereotypes.* Unpublished manuscript, University of Wisconsin-Madison.

Brubaker, R. G., & Loftin, T. L. (1987). Smokeless tobacco use by middle school males: A preliminary test of the reasoned action theory. *Journal of School Health, 57,* 64-67.

Burns, D., & Pierce, J. (1992). *Tobacco use in California 1990-1991.* Sacramento: Department of Health Services.

Burnstein, L. (1980). The analysis of multilevel data in educational research and evaluation. *Review of Research in Education, 8,* 158-233.

Burton, D. (1978). Motivating smokers to assume personal responsibility for quitting. In J. L. Schwartz (Ed.), *Progress in smoking cessation.* New York: American Cancer Society/World Health Organization/Union Internationale Contre le Cancer.

Burton, D. (1994). Tobacco cessation programs for adolescents. In R. Richmond (Ed.), *Interventions for smokers: An international perspective* (pp. 95-105). Baltimore: Williams & Wilkins.

Burton, D., Chakravorty, B., Flay, B. R., Sussman, S., Dent, C. W., & Stacy, A. W. (1994). *Outcomes of a tobacco use cessation school-based clinic program: Project TNT.* Manuscript submitted for publication.

Burton, D., Sussman, S., Dent, C. W., Graham, M., & Hahn, G. (1989, October). In L. Burhansstipanov (panel presider), *Use and cessation of smokeless tobacco and cigarettes by high school students.* Panel presented at the Fortieth Annual Meeting and Conference of the Society for Public Health Education (SOPHE) Association, Chicago.

Burton, D., Sussman, S., Hansen, W. B., Johnson, C. A., & Flay B. R. (1989). Image attributions and smoking among seventh grade students. *Journal of Applied Social Psychology, 19,* 656-664.

Campanelli, P. C., Dielman, T. E., & Shope, J. T. (1987). Validity of adolescents self-reports of alcohol use and misuse using a bogus pipeline procedure. *Adolescence, 22*(85), 7-22.

Campbell, D. T., & Fiske, D. W. (1959). Convergent and discriminant validation by the multitrait-multimethod matrix. *Psychological Bulletin, 56*(2), 81-106.

Campbell, D. T., & Stanley, J. C. (1973). *Experimental and quasi-experimental designs for research.* Chicago: Rand McNally.

Charlin, V. L., Sussman, S., Dent, C. W., Stacy, A. W., Graham, J. W., Barovich, M., Hahn, G., Burton, D., & Flay, B. R. (1990). Three methods of assessing adolescent school-level experimentation of tobacco products. *Evaluation Review, 14*(3), 297-307.

Chassin, L. A., Presson, C. C., & Sherman, S. J. (1985). Stepping backward in order to step forward: An acquisition-oriented approach to primary prevention. *Journal of Consulting and Clinical Psychology, 53,* 612-622.

Chassin, L. A., Presson, C. C., & Sherman, S. J. (1990). Social psychological contributions to the understanding and prevention of adolescent cigarette smoking. *Personality and Social Psychology Bulletin, 16*(1), 133-151.

Chassin, L. A., Presson, C. C., Sherman, S. J., Corty, E., & Olshavsky, R. O. (1984). Predicting the onset of adolescent cigarettes smoking in adolescents: A longitudinal study. *Journal of Applied Social Psychology, 14*, 224-243.

Chassin, L. A., Presson, C. C., Sherman, S. J., & Margolis, S. (1988). The social image of smokeless tobacco use in the three different types of teenagers. *Addictive Behaviors, 13*, 107-112.

Chassin, L. A., Presson, C. C., Sherman, S. J., McLaughlin, L., & Goila, D. (1985). Psychosocial correlates of adolescent smokeless tobacco use. *Addictive Behaviors, 10*, 431-435.

Chen, T. T. L., & Winder, A. E. (1985). Teachers' perceptions related to smoking education between 1973 and 1982. *Journal of Drug Education, 15*, 125-137.

Christen, A. G. (1976). Candy breath mints, acidic beverages and traumatic brushing: Suspected factors in tooth erosion and abrasion. Case report. *Texas Dental Journal, 94*, 10-12.

Christen, A. G., & Swanson, B. Z. (1983). Orally used smokeless tobacco use advertised in the metaphoric trade cards of 1870-1900. *Bulletin of the History of Dentistry, 31*, 82-86.

Christenson, G. M., Gold, R. S., Katz, M., & Kreuter, M. W. (1985). Preface. Special Issue of *Journal of School Health* on the School Health Education Evaluation (SHEE), *55*(8), 295-298.

Cialdini, R. B., Reno, R. R., & Kallgren, C. A. (1990). A focus theory of normative conduct: Recycling the concept of norms to reduce littering in public places. *Journal of Personality and Social Psychology, 58*, 1015-1026.

Cinnamin, D. (1993). *An experimental test of smoking cessation clinics for continuation high school youth.* Unpublished master's thesis, California Lutheran University, Thousand Oaks.

Clarke, J. H., MacPherson, B., Holmes, D. R., & Jones, R. (1986). Reducing adolescent smoking: A comparison of peer-led, teacher-led, and expert interventions. *Journal of School Health, 56*, 102-106.

Clasen, D. R., & Brown, B. B. (1985). The multi-dimensionality of peer pressure in adolescence. *Journal of Youth and Adolescence, 14*(6), 451-468.

Cleary, M. J., & Gobble, D. (1990). The changing nature of public schools: Implications for teacher preparation. *Journal of School Health, 60*, 53-55.

Cohen, J. (1977). *Statistical power analysis for the behavioral sciences.* New York: Academic Press.

Cohen, J., & Cohen, P. (1979). *Applied multiple regression/correlation analysis for the behavioral sciences.* New York: John Wiley.

Cohen, S., Kamarck, T., & Mermelstein, R. (1983). A global measure of perceived stress. *Journal of Health and Social Behavior, 24*, 385-395.

Collins, L. M., Sussman, S., Rauch, J. M., Dent, C. W., Johnson, C. A., Hansen, W. B., & Flay, B. R. (1987). Psychosocial predictors or young adolescent cigarette smoking: A sixteen-month, three-wave longitudinal study. *Journal of Applied Social Psychology, 17*, 554-573.

Connolly, G. N., Winn, D. M. Hecht, S. S., Henningfield, J. E., Walker, B., & Hoffman, D. (1986). The reemergence of smokeless tobacco. *New England Journal of Medicine, 314*, 1020-1026.

Conrad, K. M., Flay, B. R., & Hill, D. (1992). Why children start smoking cigarettes: Predictors of onset. *British Journal of the Addictions, 87,* 1711-1724.

Cook, T. D., & Campbell, D. T. (1979). *Quasi-experimentation design and analysis issues for field settings.* Chicago: Rand McNally.

Corcoran, R. D., & Allegrante, J. P. (1989). Vocational education students: A difficult-to-reach population at risk for smoking-related cancer. *Journal of School Health, 59*(5), 195-198.

Costanzo, P. R., & Shaw, M. E. (1966). Conformity as a function of age level. *Child Development, 37,* 967-975.

Craig, S., Dent, C. W., & Sussman, S. (1988). *School selection and recruitment. Phase 1: Other major tasks, Project Towards No Tobacco Use (TNT)* (Technical Report #88-TNT-01). Los Angeles: University of Southern California: Institute for Health Promotion and Disease Prevention Research.

Crowne, D. P., & Marlowe, D. (1960). A new scale of social desirability independent of psychopathology. *Journal of Counseling Psychology, 24,* 349-354.

Custer, A., Gildea, S., & Liverman, L. (1989). *TNT Data collection* (Technical Report #89-TNT-04). Los Angeles: University of Southern California, Institute for Health Promotion and Disease Prevention Research.

DeArmas, A., & Brigham, T. A. (1986). Moderated role-play validity: Do some subjects role play more naturally than others? *Behavioral Assessment, 8,* 341-347.

Del Greco, L. (1980). Assertion training to prevent adolescent cigarette smoking. *Health Education Journal, 39,* 80-83.

DeMoor, C., Elder, J. P., Young, R. L., Wildey, M. B., & Molgaard, C. A. (1989). Generic tobacco use among four ethnic groups in a school age population. *Journal of Drug Education, 19*(3), 257-270.

Dent, C. W. (1988). *Using SAS linear models to assess and correct for attrition bias.* Paper presented at the 13th Annual Conference of SAS User's Group International, Orlando, FL.

Dent, C. W. (1989). *Random assignment in Project TNT and data collection procedures* (Technical Report #89-TNT-01). Los Angeles: University of Southern California, Institute for Health Promotion and Disease Prevention Research.

Dent, C. W., Galaif, J., Sussman, S., Stacy, A. W., Burton, D., & Flay, B. R. (1993). Demographic, psychosocial and behavioral differences in sample of actively and passively consented adolescents. *Addictive Behaviors, 18,* 51-56.

Dent, C. W., & Sussman, S. (1990, December). *A comparison of complete and partial sampling in repeatedly accessible populations of naturally clustered units.* Paper presented at the Symposium on Statistical Methods for Evaluation of Intervention and Prevention Strategies, Atlanta.

Dent, C. W., Sussman, S., & Flay, B. R. (1993). The use of archival data to select and assign schools in a drug prevention trial. *Evaluation Review, 17*(2), 159-181.

Dent, C. W., Sussman, S., Johnson, C. A., Hansen, W. B., & Flay, B. R. (1987). Adolescent smokeless tobacco incidence: Relations with other drugs and psychosocial variables. *Preventive Medicine, 16,* 422-431.

Dent, C. W., Sussman, S., Stacy, A. W., Burton, D., & Flay, B. R. (in preparation). Biochemical validation of self-reports of tobacco use: Is there an advantage of cotinine versus CO measures?

Dent, C. W., Sussman, S., Stacy, A. W., Craig, S., Burton, D., & Flay, B. R. (1994). *Project Towards No Tobacco Use: Two-year behavior outcomes.* Manuscript submitted for publication.

Deutsch, M., & Gerard, H. B. (1955). A study of normative and informational social influences upon individual judgment. *Journal of Abnormal and Social Psychology, 51*, 629-636.

Devine, P. G., & Ostrom, T. M. (1988). Dimensional versus information-processing approaches to social knowledge: The case of inconsistency management. In D. Bartal & A. W. Kruglanski (Eds.), *The social psychology of knowledge* (pp. 231-261). Cambridge, UK: Cambridge University Press.

DiLorenzo, T. M., Kern, T. G., & Pieper, R. M. (1991). Treatment of smokeless tobacco use through a formalized cessation program. *Behavior Therapy, 22*, 41-46.

Donner, A. (1982). An empirical study of cluster randomization. *International Journal of Epidemiology, 11*, 283-286.

Donner, A. (1985). A regression approach to the analysis of data arising from cluster randomization. *International Journal of Epidemiology, 14*, 322-326.

Donovan, J. E., & Jessor, R. (1985). Structure of problem behavior in adolescence and young adulthood. *Journal of Consulting and Clinical Psychology, 53*, 890-904.

Dunphy, D. C. (1963). The social structure of urban adolescent peer groups. *Sociometry, 26*, 230-246.

Dwyer, J. H. (1983). *Statistical models for the social and behavioral sciences.* New York: Oxford University Press.

Eakin, E., Severson, H., & Glasgow, R. E. (1989). Development and evaluation of a smokeless tobacco cessation program: A pilot study. *National Cancer Institute Monographs, 95*, 95-100.

Eckert, P. (1983). Beyond the statistics of adolescent smoking. *American Journal of Public Health, 73*, 439-441.

Eckert, P. (1989). *Jocks and burnouts: Social categories and identity in the high school.* New York: Teachers College Press.

Edmundson, E. W., Glover, E. D., Holbert, D., Alston, P. P., & Schroeder, K. L. (1988). Personality profiles associated with smokeless tobacco use patterns. *Addictive Behaviors, 13*, 219-223.

Eiseman, S., Robinson, J., & Zapata, M. D. A. (1984). Disciplinary approach for teacher effectiveness training in drug education. *Journal of Drug Education, 14*, 357-367.

Eiser, J. R. (1980). *Cognitive social psychology: A guidebook to theory and research.* Maidenhead, UK: McGraw-Hill.

Eiser, J. R. (1985). Smoking: The social learning of an addiction. *Journal of Social and Clinical Psychology, 3*, 446-457.

Elder, J. P., & Stern, R. A. (1986). The ABCs of adolescent smoking prevention: An environment and skills model. *Health Education Quarterly, 13*, 181-191.

Elder, J. P., Wildey, M., de Moor, C., Sallis, J. F., Eckhardt, L., Edwards, C., Erickson, A., Golbeck, A., Hovell, M., Johnston, D., Levitz, M. D., Molgaard, C., Young, R., Vito, D., & Woodruff, S. I. (1993). The long-term prevention of tobacco use among junior high school students: Classroom and telephone interventions. *American Journal of Public Health, 83*, 1239-1244.

Erickson, E. H. (1968). *Identity, youth and crisis.* New York: Norton.

Ernster, V. L. (1989). Advertising and promotion of smokeless tobacco products. *National Cancer Institute Monographs, 8*, 87-94.

Evans, R. I. (1976). Smoking in children: Developing a social psychological strategy of deterrence. *Preventive Medicine, 5*, 122-127.

Evans, R. I. (1988). Health promotion-science or idealogy? *Health Psychology, 7*(3), 203-219.

Evans, R. I., Hansen, W. B., & Mittelmark, M. B. (1977). Increasing the validity of self-reports of smoking behavior in children. *Journal of Applied Social Psychology, 62*(4), 521-523.

Evans, R. I., Henderson, A., Hill, P., & Raines, B. (1979). Smoking in children and adolescents: Psychosocial determinants and prevention strategies. In N. A. Krasnegor (Ed.), *The behavioral aspects of smoking* (NIDA Research Monograph 26) (pp. 69-96). Rockville, MD: National Institute on Drug Abuse.

Evans, R. I., Raines, B. E., & Owen, A. E. (1989). Formative evaluation in school-based health promotion investigations. *Preventive Medicine, 18,* 229-234.

Evans, R. I., Rozelle, R. M., Mittelmark, M. B., Hansen, W. B., Bane, A. L., & Havis, J. (1978). Deterring the onset of smoking in children: Knowledge of immediate physiological effects and coping with peer pressure, media pressure, and parent modeling. *Journal of Applied Social Psychology, 8*(2), 126-135.

Feldman, J. M., & Lynch, J. G. (1988). Self-generated validity and other effects of measurement on belief, attitude, intention, and behavior. *Journal of Applied Psychology, 73,* 421-435.

Festinger, L. (1954). A theory of social comparison processes. *Human Relations, 7,* 177-140.

Fielding, J. E., & Phenow, K. J. (1988). Health effects of involuntary smoking. *New England Journal of Medicine, 319,* 1452-1460.

Fincher, J. (1985, October). Sean Marsee's smokeless death. *Readers Digest, 127*(76) 107-112.

Fishbein, M. (1982). Social psychological analysis of smoking behavior. In J. R. Eiser (Ed.), *Social psychology and behavioral medicine* (pp. 179-197). Manchester, UK: John Wiley.

Fishkin, S. A., Sussman, S., Stacy, A. W., Dent, C. W., Burton, D., & Flay, B. R. (1993). Ingroup versus outgroup perceptions of the characteristics of high-risk youth: Negative stereotyping. *Journal of Applied Social Psychology, 23*(13), 1051-1068.

Flay, B. R. (1981). Evaluation of mass media prevention campaigns. In R. R. Rice & W. J. Paisley (Eds.), *Public communications campaigns* (pp. 239-313). Beverly Hills, CA: Sage.

Flay, B. R. (1985). Psychosocial approaches to smoking prevention: A review of findings. *Health Psychology, 4,*(5), 449-488.

Flay, B. R. (1986). Efficacy and effectiveness trials (and other phases of research) in the development of health promotion programs. *Preventive Medicine, 15,* 451-474.

Flay, B. R. (1987a). Social psychological approaches to smoking prevention: Review and recommendations. *Advances in Health Education and Promotion, 2,* 121-180.

Flay, B. R. (1987b). Mass media and smoking cessation: A critical review. *American Journal of Public Health, 76,* 153-160.

Flay, B. R., & Best, J. A. (1982). Overcoming design problems in the evaluation of health behavior change programs. *Evaluation and the Health Professions, 5,* 43-69.

Flay, B. R., Brannon, B. R., Johnson, C. A., Hansen, W. B., Ulene, A. L., Whitney-Saltiel, D. A., Gleason, L. R., Sussman, S., Gavin, M., Glowacz, K. M., & Sobol, D. F. (1988). The television, school, and family smoking prevention/cessation project: I. Theoretical basis and television program development. *Preventive Medicine, 17,* 585-607.

Flay, B. R., d'Avernas, J. R., Best, J. A., Kersall, M. W., & Ryan, K. B. (1983). Cigarette smoking: Why young people do it and ways of preventing it: The Waterloo

Study. In P. Firestone & P. McGrath (Eds.), *Pediatric and adolescent behavioral medicine* (pp. 132-183). New York: Springer-Verlag.

Flay, B. R., Koepke, D., Thompson, S. J., Santi, S., Best, J. A., & Brown, K. S. (1989). Six-year followup of the first Waterloo School Smoking Prevention Trial. *American Journal of Public Health, 79,* 1371-1380.

Flay, B. R., Ryan, K. B., Best, J. A., Brown, K. S., Kersell, M. W., d'Avernas, J. R., & Zanna, M. P. (1985). Are social-psychological smoking prevention programs effective? The Waterloo Study. *Journal of Behavioral Medicine, 8,* 37-59.

Forster, J. L., Klepp, K. I., & Jeffery, R. W. (1989). Sources of cigarettes for tenth graders in two Minnesota cities. *Health Education Research: Theory and Practice, 4,* 45-50.

Franco, D. P., Chistoff, K. A., Crimmins, D. B., & Kelly, J. A. (1983). Social skills training for an extremely shy young adolescent: An empirical case study. *Behavioral Therapy, 14,* 568-575.

Freier, M. C., Bell, R. M., & Ellickson, P. L. (1991). *Do teens tell the truth? The validity of self-reported tobacco use by adolescents* (RAND Note #N-3291-CHF). Santa Monica, CA: RAND.

Friedman, L. S., Lichtenstein, E., & Biglan, A. (1985). Smoking onset among teens: A empirical analysis of initial situations. *Addictive Behaviors, 10,* 1-13.

Galaif, E. R., Sussman, S., & Bundek, N. (1994). *The relations of school staff smokers' attitudes about modeling smoking behavior in students and their receptivity to no-smoking policy.* Manuscript submitted for publication.

Gambrill, E. D., & Richey, C. A. (1975). An assertion inventory for use in assessment and research. *Behavior Therapy, 6,* 550-561.

Gavin, L. A., & Furman, W. (1989). Age differences in adolescents' perceptions of their groups. *Developmental Psychology, 25,* 827-834.

Gibbons, R. D., & Bock, R. D. (1987). Trend in correlated proportions. *Psychometrika, 52,* 113-124.

Gillies, P. A., Wilcox, B., Coates, C., Krismundsdottir, F., & Reid, D. J. (1982). Use of objective measure in the validation of self-reported smoking in children aged 10 and 11 years: Saliva thiocyanate. *Journal of Epidemiology and Community Health, 36,* 205-208.

Glasgow, R. E., & Lichtenstein, E. (1987). Long-term effects of behavioral smoking cessation interventions. *Behavior Therapy, 18,* 297-324.

Glasgow, R. E., McCaul, K. D., Freeborn, V. B., & O'Neill, H. K. (1981). Immediate and long term health consequences information in the prevention of adolescent smoking. *Behavior Therapist, 4,* 15-16.

Glover, E. D. (1986). Conducting smokeless tobacco cessation clinics. *American Journal of Public Health, 76*(2), 207.

Glover, E. D., Christen A. G., & Henderson, A. H. (1981). Smokeless tobacco and the adolescent male. *Journal of Early Adolescence, 2,* 1-13.

Glynn, K., Levanthal, H., & Hirschman, R. (1985). A cognitive developmental approach to smoking prevention. In C. S. Bell & R. Battjes (Eds.), *Prevention research: Deterring drug abuse among children and adolescents* (NIDA Research Monograph 63) (pp. 130-152). Rockville, MD: National Institute on Drug Abuse.

Glynn, S. M., Gruder, C. L., & Jegerski, J. A. (1986). Effects of biochemical validation of self- reported cigarette smoking on treatment success and on misreporting abstinence. *Health Psychology, 5*(2), 125-136.

Glynn, T. J. (1989). Essential elements of school-based smoking prevention programs. *Journal of School Health, 59*(5), 181-188.

Glynn, T. J., & Cullen, J. W. (1989). Health promotion through smoking prevention and cessation—The need for a selective research agenda. *Health Education Research: Theory and Practice, 4,* 5-12.

Goldfried, M. R., & Davison, G. C. (1976). *Clinical behavior therapy.* New York: Holt, Rinehart & Winston.

Gottlieb, B. H. (1985). Social networks and social support: An overview of research, practice, and policy implications. *Health Education Quarterly, 12,* 5-22.

Graham, J. W., & Donaldson, S. I. (1993). Evaluating interventions with differential attrition: The importance of non-response mechanisms and use of followup data. *Journal of Applied Psychology, 78*(1), 119-128.

Graham, J. W., Flay, B. R., Johnson, C. A., Hansen, W. B., & Collins, L. M. (1984). Group comparability: A multi-attribute utility approach to the use of random assignment with small numbers of aggregated units. *Evaluation Review, 8,* 247-260.

Graham, J. W., Flay, B. R., Johnson, C. A., Hansen, W. B., Grossman, L., & Sobel, J. L. (1984). Reliability of self-report measures of drug use in prevention research: Evaluation of the Project SMART questionnaire via the test-retest reliability matrix. *Journal of Drug Education, 14,* 175-193.

Graham, J. W., Johnson, C. A., Hansen, W. B., Flay, B. R., & Gee, M. (1990). Drug use prevention programs, gender, and ethnicity: Evaluation of three seventh-grade Project SMART cohorts. *Preventive Medicine, 19,* 305-313.

Graham, J. W., Marks, G., & Hansen, W. B. (1991). Social influence processes affecting adolescent substance use. *Journal of Applied Psychology, 76,* 291-298.

Graham, J. W., Rohrbach, L. A., Hansen, W. B., Flay, B. R., & Johnson, C. A. (1989). Convergent and discriminant validity for assessment of skill in resisting a role play alcohol offer. *Behavioral Assessment, 11,* 353-379.

Graham, J. W., Sobel, J. L., Grossman, L. M., Flay, B. R., Hansen, W. B., & Johnson, C. A. (1985, January). *Reliability of self-report measures in drug abuse prevention research: Evaluation of psychosocial measures in the Project SMART questionnaire* (Technical Report Series, Health Behavior Research Institute). Los Angeles: University of Southern California Press.

Graham, M., Burton, D., Flay, B. R., Hahn, G., Craig, S., Sussman, S., Dent, C., & Stacy, A. (1993). *The use of focus groups to develop motivational strategies for tobacco use cessation among high school students.* Unpublished manuscript.

Granovetter, M. (1973). The strength of weak ties. *American Journal of Sociology, 78,* 1360-1380.

Green, D. E. (1977). Psychological factors in smoking. In M. E. Jarvik, J. W. Cullen, E. R. Gritz, T. M. Vogt, & L. J. West (Eds.), *Research on smoking behavior* (pp. 149-156). Rockville, MD: National Institute on Drug Abuse, Public Health Service, Department of Health, Education and Welfare.

Green, D. E. (1979). *Teenage smoking: Immediate and long-term patterns.* Washington, DC: National Institute of Education.

Greenberg, R. A., Bauman, K. E., Strecher, V. J., Keyes, L. L., Glover, L. H., Haley, N. J., Stedman, H. C., & Loda, F. A. (1991). Passive smoking during the first year of life. *American Journal of Public Health, 81,* 850-853.

Gritz, E. R., Baer-Weiss, V., Benowitz, N. L., Van Vunakis, H., & Jarvik, M. E. (1981). Plasma nicotine and cotinine concentrations in habitual smokeless tobacco users. *Clinical Pharmacological Therapy, 30,* 201-209.

Gritz, E. R., Ksir, C., & McCarthy, W. J. (1985). Smokeless tobacco use in the United States: Present and future trends. *Annals of Behavioral Medicine, 2,* 24-27.

Haas, A. P., Hendin, H., & Singer, P. (1987). Psychodynamic and structural interviewing: Issues of validity. *Comprehensive Psychiatry, 28*(1), 40-53.

Hahn, G., Charlin, V., Sussman, S., Manzi, J., Dent, C. W., Stacy, A., Burton, D., Flay, B. R., & Hansen, W. B. (1990). Adolescents' first and last use situations of smokeless tobacco and cigarettes: Similarities and differences. *Addictive Behaviors, 15*, 439-448.

Hahn, G., Craig, S., Abrams, C., Barovich, M., Selski, E., & Sussman, S. (1989). *Project Towards No Tobacco Use (TNT): Tobacco use prevention guide, physical consequences curriculum.* Los Angeles: University of Southern California, Institute for Health Promotion and Disease Prevention Research.

Haley, N. J., Axelrod, C. M., & Tilton, K. A. (1983). Validation of self-reported smoking behavior: Biochemical analyses of cotinine and thiocyanate. *American Journal of Public Health, 73*, 1204-1207.

Hall, A., & Wellman, B. (1985). Social networks and social support. In S. Cohen & S. L. Syme (Eds.), *Social Support and Health* (pp. 23-42). New York: Academic Press.

Hansen, W. B., Collins, L. M., Johnson, C. A., & Graham, J. W. (1985). Self-initiated smoking cessation among high school students. *Addictive Behaviors, 10*, 265-271.

Hansen, W. B., Collins, L. M., Malotte, C. K., Johnson, C. A., & Fielding, J. E. (1985). Attrition in prevention research. *Journal of Behavioral Medicine, 8*, 261-275.

Hansen, W. B., & Graham, J. W. (1991). Preventing alcohol, marijuana, and cigarette use among adolescents: Peer pressure resistance training versus establishing conservative norms. *Preventive Medicine, 20*, 414-430.

Hansen, W. B., Graham, J. W., Wolkenstein, B. H., Lundy, B. Z., Pearson, J. L., Flay, B. R., & Johnson, C. A. (1988). Differential impact of three alcohol prevention curricula on hypothesized mediating variables. *Journal of Drug Education, 18*, 143-153.

Hansen, W. B., Johnson, C. A., Flay, B. R., Graham, J. W., & Sobel, J. (1988). Affective and social influences approaches to the prevention of multiple substance abuse among seventh grade students: Results from Project SMART. *Preventive Medicine, 17*, 135-154.

Hansen, W. B., & Mallotte, K. C. (1986). Perceived personal immunity: The development of beliefs about susceptibility to the consequences of smoking. *Preventive Medicine, 15*, 363-372.

Hansen, W. B., Mallotte, K. C., & Fielding, J. E. (1985). The bogus pipeline revisited: The use of the threat as a means of increasing self-reports of tobacco use. *Journal of Applied Psychology, 70*,(4), 789-792.

Hartup, W., & Louge, R. (1979). Peers as models. *School Psychology Digest, 4*, 11-21.

Headen, S. W., Bauman, K. E., Deane, G. D., & Koch, G. G. (1991). Are the correlates of cigarette smoking initiation different for black and white adolescents? *American Journal of Public Health, 81*, 854-857.

Heckman, J. J. (1979). Sample selection bias as a specification error. *Econometrica, 47*, 153-161.

Hedeker, D., Gibbons, R. D., & Flay, B. R. (1994). *Random regression models for clustered data: With an example from smoking prevention research.* Manuscript submitted for publication.

Heimann-Ratain, G., Hanson, M., & Peregoy, S. M. (1985). The role of focus group interviews in designing a smoking prevention program. *Journal of School Health, 55*, 13-16.

Hendricks, C. M., Echols, D., & Nelson, G. D. (1989). The impact of a preschool health curriculum on children's health knowledge. *Journal of School Health, 59*(9), 389-395.

Henningfield, J. E. (1986). Evidence that smokeless tobacco use may lead to dependence. In *NIH Consensus Development Conference: Health implications of smokeless tobacco and abstracts*. Bethesda, MD: National Institutes of Health.

Hetherington, E., & Parke, R. D. (1975). *Child psychology: A contemporary viewpoint*. New York: McGraw-Hill.

Higgins, I.T.T., Mahan, C. M., & Wynder, E. L. (1988). Lung cancer among cigar and pipe smokers. *Preventive Medicine, 17*, 117-128.

Hilliard, A.S.A. (1976). *Alternatives to IQ testing: An approach to the identification of gifted minority children. Final report to the California State Department of Education*.

Hirschman, R. S., Leventhal, H., Fleming, R., & Glynn, K. (1987, August). *A cognitive-developmental program to prevent smoking*. Paper presented at the 95th Annual Convention of the American Psychological Association, New York.

Holcomb, J. D., Nelson, J., Carbonari, J., Ingersoll, R. W., Chamberlain, R. M., Luce, W. M., & Weinberg, A. D. (1984). Integrating cardiovascular health education with an English curriculum in a secondary school. *Journal of School Health, 54*, 339-342.

Hops, H., Weissman, W., Biglan, A., Thompson, R., Faller, C., & Severson, H. H. (1986). A taped situation test of cigarette refusal skill among adolescents. *Behavioral Assessment, 8*, 145-154.

Hu, B. (in preparation). Use of smokeless tobacco and the unidimensional model of drug involvement.

Hunter, S. M., Croft, J. B., Burke, G. L., Parker, F. C., Webber, L. S., & Berenson, G. S. (1986). Longitudinal patterns of cigarette smoking and smokeless tobacco use in youth: The Bogalusa Heart Study. *American Journal of Public Health, 76*, 193-195.

Hurd, P. D., Johnson, C. A., Pechacek, T., Bast, L. P., Jacobs, D. R., & Luepker, R. V. (1980). Prevention of cigarette smoking in seventh grade students. *Journal of Behavioral Medicine, 3*(1), 15-28.

Jessor, R. (1984). Adolescent development and behavioral health. In J. D. Matarazzo, S. M. Weiss, J. A. Herd, N. E. Miller, & S. M. Weiss (Eds), *Behavioral health: A handbook of health enhancement and disease prevention* (pp. 69-90). New York: John Wiley.

Jessor, R., & Jessor, S. L. (1977). *Problem behavior and psychosocial development: A longitudinal study of youth*. New York: Academic Press.

Johnson, B. D. (1980). Toward a theory of drug subcultures. In D. J. Lettieu, M. Sayers, & H. W. Peerson (Eds.), *Theories on drug abuse* (NIDA Research Monograph 30) (pp. 110-119). Rockville, MD: National Institute on Drug Abuse.

Johnson, C. A. (1981). Untested and erroneous assumptions underlying anti-smoking programs. In T. Coates, A. Peterson, & C. Perry (Eds.), *Promotion of health in youth* (chap. 9). New York: Academic Press.

Johnson, C. A. (1986). Prevention and control of drug abuse. In J. M. Last (Ed.), *Maxcy-Rosenam public health and preventive medicine* (12th ed., pp. 1075-1087). Norwalk, CT: Appleton-Century-Crofts.

Johnson, C. A., Dent, C. W., Sussman, S., & Sanford, D. (September, 1993). *Countermanding social and advertising influences on youth to smoke*. Paper presentation at the American Cancer Society's Workshop on Children with Cancer, Naples, Florida.

Johnson, C. A., Hansen, W. B., Collins, L. M., & Graham, W. B. (1986). High-school smoking prevention: Results of a three-year longitudinal study. *Journal of Behavioral Medicine, 9*, 439-452.

Johnson, C. A., Pentz, M. A., Weber, M. D., Dwyer, J. H., Baer, N., MacKinnon, D. P., Hansen, W. B., & Flay, B. R. (1990). Relative effectiveness of comprehensive community programming for drug abuse prevention with high-risk and low-risk adolescents. *Journal of Consulting and Clinical Psychology, 58,* 447-456.

Johnston, L. D., O'Malley, P. M., & Bachman, J. G. (1993). *National survey results on drug use from the monitoring the future study, 1975-1992: Vol. 1. Secondary School Students.* Rockville, MD: National Institute on Drug Abuse.

Jones, C. J., Schiffman, M. H., Kurman, R., Jacob, P., & Benowitz, N. L. (1991). Elevated nicotine levels in cervical lavages from passive smokers. *American Journal of Public Health, 81,* 378-379.

Jones, E. E. (1964). *Ingratiation: A social analysis.* New York: Appelton-Century-Crofts.

Jones, E. E., Kanouse, D. E., Kelley, H. H., Nisbett, R. E., Valins, S., & Weiner, B. (1972). *Attribution: Perceiving the causes of behavior.* Morristown, NJ: General Learning Press.

Jones, E. E., & Sigall, L. (1971). The bogus pipeline: A new paradigm for measuring affect and attitude. *Psychological Bulletin, 76,* 349-364.

Jones, E. E., & Wortman, C. (1973). *Ingratiation: An attributed approach.* Morristown, NJ: General Learning Press.

Jones, R. B. (1987). Use of smokeless tobacco in the 1986 World Series. *New England Journal of Medicine, 314,* 952.

Jones, R. R., Reid, J. B., & Patterson, G. R. (1975). Naturalistic observation in clinical assessment. In P. McReynolds (Ed.), *Advances in psychological assessment* (Vol. 3, pp. 42-95). San Francisco: Jossey-Bass.

Judd, C. M., & Kenny, D. A. (1981). Process analysis: Estimating mediation in treatment evaluations. *Evaluation Review, 5,* 602-619.

Kaplan, R. M. (1984). The connection between clinical health promotion and health status: A critical overview. *American Psychologist, 39,* 755-765.

Kazdin, A. E., & Wilcoxon, L. A. (1976). Systematic desensitization and nonspecific treatment effects: A methodological evaluation. *Psychological Bulletin, 83,* 729-753.

Kelley, H. H. (1952). Two functions of reference groups. In G. E. Swanson, T. M. Newcomb, & E. L. Hartley (Eds.), *Readings in social psychology* (pp. 410-414). New York: Holt, Rinehart, & Winston.

Kelly, J. A. (1982). *Social-skills training: A practical guide for interventions.* New York: Springer.

Kenton, C., & Blot, W. J. (1986). *National Library of Medicine literature search: Health effects of smokeless tobacco use.* Bethesda, MD: National Institutes of Health.

Kidder, L. H. (1981). *Research methods in social relations* (4th ed.). New York: Holt, Rinehart & Winston.

Kiesler, C. A. (1971). *The psychology of commitment: Experiments linking behavior to beliefs.* New York: Academic Press.

Kiesler, C. A., & Kiesler, S. R. (1970). *Conformity.* Reading, MA: Addison-Wesley.

Kirn, T. F. (1987). Laws ban minors' tobacco purchases, but enforcement is another matter. *Journal of the American Medical Association, 257*(24), 3323-3324.

Kliebard, H. M. (1989). Problems of definition in curriculum. *Journal of Curriculum and Supervision, 5*(1), 1-5.

Koepke, D., & Flay, B. R. (1989). Levels of analysis. In M. T. Braverman (Ed.), *Evaluating health promotion programs* (New Directions for Program Evaluation No. 43) (pp. 75-87). San Francisco: Jossey-Bass.

Koepke, D., Flay, B. R., & Johnson, C. A. (1990). Health behaviors in minority families: The case of cigarette smoking. *Family Community Health, 13*(1), 35-43.

Koop, C. E. (1986). The quest for a smoke-free young America by the year 2000. *Journal of School Health, 56*, 8-12.

Kristiansen, C. M. (1986). A two-value model of preventive health behavior. *Basic and Applied Social Psychology, 7*, 173-184.

Krosnick, J. A., & Judd, C. M. (1982). Transitions in social influence at adolescence: Who induces cigarette smoking? *Developmental Psychology, 18*(3), 359-368.

Krueger, R. A. (1988). *Focus groups: A practical guide for applied research.* Newbury Park, CA: Sage.

Kunstel, F. (1978). Assessing community needs: Implications for curriculum and staff development in health education. *Journal of School Health, 48*(4), 220-224.

Larkin, J. E. (1987). Are good teachers perceived as high self-monitors? *Personality and Social Psychology Bulletin, 13*, 64-72.

Larkin, R. W. (1979). *Suburban youth in cultural crisis.* New York: Oxford University Press.

Leventhal, H., & Cleary, P. D. (1980). The smoking problem: A review of the research and theory in behavioral risk modification. *Psychological Bulletin, 88*, 370-405.

Leventhal, H., Glynn, K., & Fleming, R. (1987). Is the smoking decision an 'informed choice'? Effect of smoking risk factors on smoking beliefs. *Journal of the American Medical Association, 257*(24), 3373-3376.

Lewis, C. E., & Lewis, M. A. (1984). Peer pressure and risk-taking behaviors in children. *American Journal of Public Health, 74*, 580-584.

Lichtenstein, E. (1982). The smoking problem: A behavioral perspective. *Journal of Consulting and Clinical Psychology, 50*(6), 804-819.

Lichtenstein, E., & Glasgow, R. E. (1992). Smoking cessation: What have we learned over the past decade? *Journal of Consulting and Clinical Psychology, 4*, 518-527.

Lichtenstein, E., & Mermelstein, R. J. (1984). Review of approaches to smoking treatment: Behavior modification strategies. In J. D. Matarazzo, S. M. Weiss, J. A. Herd, N. E. Miller, & L.S.M. Weiss (Eds.), *Behavioral health* (pp. 695-712). New York: John Wiley.

Lichtenstein, E., Severson, H. H., Friedman, L. S., & Ary, D. V. (1984). Chewing tobacco use by adolescents: Prevalence in relation to cigarette smoking. *Addictive Behaviors, 9*, 351-355.

Linn, M. W., & Stein, S. (1985). Reasons for smoking among extremely heavy smokers. *Addictive Behaviors, 10*, 197-201.

Lofland, J. (1971). *Analyzing social settings.* Belmont, CA: Wadsworth.

Lopes, C., Sussman, S., Galaif, E. R., & Crippens, D. L. (in press). The impact of a videotape on smoking cessation among African-American women. *American Journal of Health Promotion.*

Lotecka, L. L., & MacWhinney, M. (1983). Enhancing decision behavior in high school "smokers." *International Journal of the Addictions, 18*, 479-490.

Lubinski, D., & Humphreys, L. G. (1990). Assessing spurious "moderator effects": Illustrated substantively with the hypothesized ("synergistic") relation between spatial and mathematical ability. *Psychological Bulletin, 107*, 385-393.

Luepker, R. V., Johnson, C. A., Murray, D. M., & Pechacek, T. F. (1983). Prevention of cigarette smoking: Three-year follow-up of an education program for youth. *Journal of Behavioral Medicine, 6*, 53-62.

Luepker, R. V., Pechacek, T. F., Murray, D. M., Johnson, C. A., Hund, F., & Jacobs, D. R. (1981). Saliva thiocyanate: A chemical indicator of cigarette smoking in adolescents. *American Journal of Public Health, 71*, 12, 1320-1324.

MacKinnon, D. P., & Dwyer, J. H. (1993). Estimating mediated effects in prevention studies. *Evaluation Review, 17*, 144-158.

MacKinnon, D. P., Johnson, C. A., Pentz, M. A., Dwyer, J. H., & Hansen, W. B., Flay, B. R., & Wang, E.Y.I. (1991). Mediating mechanisms in a school-based drug prevention program: First year effects of the Midwestern Prevention Project. *Health Psychology, 10*, 164-172.

Marcus, A. C., Crane, L. A., Shopland, D. R., & Lynn, W. R. (1989). Use of smokeless tobacco in the United States: Recent estimates from the current population survey. *National Cancer Institute Monographs, 8*, 17-23.

Marlatt, G. A., & Gordon, N. (Eds.). (1985). *Relapse prevention.* New York: Guilford.

McAlister, A. L. (1983). Social psychological approaches. In T. J. Glynn, C. G. Leukefeld, & J. P. Ludford (Eds.), *Preventing adolescent drug abuse: Intervention strategies* (NIDA Research Monograph 47) (pp. 36-50). Rockville, MD: National Institute on Drug Abuse.

McCandless, B. R., & Koop, R. H. (1979). *Adolescents: behavior and development.* New York: Holt, Rinehart & Winston.

McCarthy, W. J. (1985). The cognitive developmental model and other alternative to the social skills deficit model of smoking onset. In C. S. Bell & R. Battjes (Eds.), *Prevention research: Deterring drug abuse among children and adolescents* (NIDA Research Monograph 63). Rockville, MD: National Institute on Drug Abuse.

McCaul, K. D., & Glasgow, R. E. (1985). Preventing adolescent smoking: What have we learned about treatment construct validity? *Health Psychology, 4*, 361-387.

McGuire, W. J. (1964). Inducing resistance to persuasion. In L. Berkowitz (Ed.), *Advances in experimental social psychology* (pp. 191-229). New York: Academic Press.

McGuire, W. J. (1969). The nature of attitude and attitude change. In G. Lindzay & E. Aronson (Eds.), *Handbook of social psychology* (2nd ed., Vol. 3, pp. 136-314). Reading, MA: Addison-Wesley.

McLaughlin, J., & Owen, S. L. (1987). Qualitative evaluation issues in funded school health projects. *Journal of School Health, 57*, 119-121.

McMorrow, M. J., & Fox, R. M. (1983). Nicotine's role in smoking: An analysis of nicotine regulation. *Psychological Bulletin, 27*, 302-327.

McNeill, A. D., Jarvis, M. J., Stapleton, J. A., Russell, M. A. H., Eiser, J. R., Gammage, P., & Gray, E. M. (1988). Prospective study of factors predicting uptake of smoking in adolescents. *Journal of Epidemiology and Community Health, 43*, 72-78.

Meichenbaum, D. (1977). *Cognitive behavior modification: An integrative approach.* New York: Plenum.

Meichenbaum, D. (1985). *Stress inoculation training.* New York: Pergamon.

Miles, M. B. (1981). *Learning to work in groups: A practical guide for members and trainers.* New York: Columbia University, Teachers College Press.

Morgan, D. L. (1988). *Focus groups as qualitative research.* Newbury Park, CA: Sage.

Mosbach, P., & Leventhal, H. (1988). Peer group identification and smoking: Implications for intervention. *Journal of Abnormal Psychology, 97*, 238-245.

Murray, D. M., O'Connell, C. M., Schmidt, L. A., & Perry, C. L. (1987). The validity of smoking self-reports by adolescents: A reexamination of the bogus pipeline procedures. *Addictive Behaviors, 12*, 7-15.

Murray, D. M., & Perry, C. L. (1987). The measurement of substance use among adolescents. When is the "bogus pipeline" method needed? *Addictive Behaviors, 12,* 225-233.

Murray, D. M., Pirie, P., Luepker, R. V., & Pallonen, U. (1989). Five and six-year follow-up results from four seventh grade smoking prevention strategies. *Journal of Behavioral Medicine, 12,* 207-218.

Murray, M., Kiryluk, S., & Swan, A. V. (1984). School characteristics and adolescent smoking: Results from the MRC/Derbyshire Smoking Study 1974-8 and from a follow-up in 1981. *Journal of Epidemiology and Community Health, 38,* 167-172.

Murray, R. P., Connett, J. E., Lauger, G. G., & Voelker, H. T. (1993). Error in smoking measures: Effects of intervention on relations of cotinine and carbon monoxide to self-reported smoking. *American Journal of Public Health, 83,* 1251-1257.

Nelson, G. D., Floyd, S., & Kolbe, L. J. (1991). Introduction: Teenage health teaching modules evaluation. *Journal of School Health, 61,* 4.

Newman, B., & Gillies, P. (1984). Methodological considerations in smoking research with children and adolescents. *Journal for the Royal Society of Health, 6,* 229-232.

Newman, I. M. (1984). Capturing the energy of peer pressure: Insights from a longitudinal study of adolescent cigarette smoking. *Journal of School Health, 54,* 146-148.

Nisbett, R. E., & Wilson, T. D. (1977). Telling more than we can know: Verbal reports on mental processes. *Psychological Review, 84,* 231-259.

Novotny, T. E., Pierce, J. P., Fiore, M. C., & Davis, R. M. (1989). Smokeless tobacco use in the United States: The adult use of tobacco surveys. *National Cancer Institute Monographs, 8,* 25-28.

Novotny, T. E., Romano, R. A., Davis, R. M., & Mills, S. L. (1992). The public health practice of tobacco control: Lessons learned and directions for the states in the 1990's. *Annual Review of Public Health, 13,* 287-318.

Nutbeam, D. (1987). Smoking among primary and secondary schoolteachers. *Health Education Journal, 46,* 14-18.

O'Leary, K. O., & Wilson, G. T. (1975). *Behavior therapy: Application and outcome.* Englewood Cliffs, NJ: Prentice Hall.

O'Neill, H. K., Glasgow, R. E., & McCaul, K. D. (1983). Component analysis in smoking prevention research: Effects of social consequences information. *Addictive Behaviors, 8,* 419-423.

Orleans, C. T., Stecher, V. J., Schoenbach, V. J., Salmon, M. A., & Blackmon, C. (1989). Smoking cessation initiatives for black Americans: Recommendations for research and intervention. *Health Education Research: Theory and Practice, 4*(1), 13-25.

Ostrom, T. M. (1990). The maturing of social cognition. In T. K. Scrull & R. S. Wyer, Jr. (Eds), *Advances in social cognition: Vol. 3. Content and process specificity in the effects of prior experiences* (pp. 153-162). Hillsdale, NJ: Lawrence Erlbaum.

Ostrom, T. M., & Upshaw, H. S. (1968). Psychological perspective and in attitude change. In A. G. Greenwald, T. C. Brook, & T. M. Ostrom (Eds.), *Psychology foundations of attitudes.* New York: Academic Press.

Pallonen, U. E. (1987). *Smoking cessation in adolescence.* Unpublished review of the literature.

Pallonen, U. E., Murray, D. M., Schmid, L., Pirie, P., & Luepker, R. V. (1990). Patterns of self-initiated smoking cessation among young adults. *Health Psychology, 9*(4), 418-426.

Pallonen, U. E., Rossi, J. S., Smith, N. F., Prochaska, J. O., & Almeida, P. M. (1993, March). *Applying the stages of change and processes of change concepts to adolescent smoking cessation.* Poster presentation at the Society of Behavioral Medicine, Fourteenth Annual Scientific Sessions, San Francisco.

Palmer, A. B. (1970). Some variables contributing to the onset of cigarette smoking in junior high school students. *Social Science and Medicine, 4,* 359-366.

Parcel, G. S., Eriksen, M. P., Lovato, C. Y., Gottlieb, N. H., Brink, S. G., & Green, L. W. (1989). The diffusion of school-based tobacco-use prevention programs: Project description and baseline data. *Health Education Research: Theory and Practice, 4,* 111-124.

Parker, V. C., & Sussman, S. (1994). *Cigarette smoking among family and friends of urban African-American youth.* Manuscript submitted for publication.

Parker, V. C., Sussman, S., Crippens, D. L., Scholl, D., Elder, P., Herring, D., & Lopes, C. E. (1994). *Use of focus groups for smoking prevention program development among urban minorities.* Manuscript submitted for publication.

Paul, G. L. (1966). *Insight versus desensitization in psychotherapy: An experiment in anxiety reduction.* Stanford, CA: Stanford University Press.

Pechacek, T. F., & Danaher, B. G. (1979). How and why people quit smoking: a cognitive-behavioral analysis. In P. C. Kendall & S. D. Hollon (Eds.), *Cognitive-behavioral interventions: Theory, research, and procedures* (pp. 389-422). New York: Academic Press.

Pechacek, T. F., Fox, B. F., Murray, D. M., & Luepker, R. V. (1984). Review of techniques for measurement of smoking behavior. In J. D. Matarazzo, S. M. Weiss, J. A. Herd, N. E. Miller, & S. M. Weiss (Eds.), *Behavioral health: A handbook of health enhancement and disease prevention* (pp. 729-754). New York: John Wiley.

Pentz, M. A. (1986). Community organization and school liaisons: How to get programs started. *Journal of School Health, 56,* 382-388.

Pentz, M. A., Brannon, B. R., Charlin, V. L., Barrett, E. J., MacKinnon, D. P., & Flay, B. R. (1989). The power of policy: Relationship of school smoking policy to adolescent smoking. *American Journal of Public Health, 79,* 857-863.

Pentz, M. A., Dwyer, J. H., MacKinnon, D. P., Flay, B. R., Hansen, W. B., Wang, E., & Johnson, C. A. (1989). A multi-community trial for primary prevention of adolescent drug abuse: Effects on drug use prevalence. *Journal of the American Medical Association, 261*(22), 3259-3266.

Pentz, M. A., Trebow, E. A., Hansen, W. B., MacKinnon, D. P., Dwyer, J. H., Johnson, C. A., Flay, B. R., Daniels, S., & Cormack, C. (1990). Effects of program implementation on adolescent drug use behavior. *Evaluation Review, 14,* 264-289.

Perry, C. L., & Jessor, R. (1983). Doing the cube: Preventing drug abuse through adolescent health promotion. In T. J. Glynn, C. G. Leukefeld, & J. P. Ludford (Eds.), *Preventing adolescent drug abuse: Intervention strategies* (NIDA Research Monograph 47) (pp. 51-75). Rockville, MD: National Institute on Drug Abuse.

Perry, C. L., Killen, J., Telch, M., Stinkard, L. A., & Danaher, B. G. (1980). Modifying smoking behavior of teenagers: A school based intervention. *American Journal of Public Health, 70* (7), 722-725.

Perry, C. L., Telch, M. J., Killen, J., Burke, R., & Maccoby, N. (1983). High school smoking prevention: The relative efficacy of varied treatments and instructions. *Adolescence, 18,* 561-566.

Petraitis, J., Flay, B. R., & Miller, T. (1994). *Substance use and the theory of triadic influence: A review and rapprochement of multivariate theories.* Manuscript submitted for publication.

Pierce, J. P. (1989). International comparisons of trends in cigarette smoking prevalence. *American Journal of Public Health. 79*(2), 1-6.

Pierce, J. P., Gilpin, E., Burns, D. M., Whalen, E., Rosbrook, B., Shopland, D., & Johnson, M. (1991). Does tobacco advertising target young people to start smoking. *Journal of the American Medical Association, 266,* 3154-3158.

Pollin, W. (1985). Addiction is the key step in causation of all tobacco-related diseases. In *Proceedings of the Seventh World Conference on Smoking and Health.* New York: American Cancer Society.

Prochaska, J. O., & DiClemente, C. C. (1983). Stages and process of self-change of smoking: Toward an integrative model of change. *Journal of Consulting and Clinical Psychology, 51*(3), 390-395.

Rathje, W. L., & Ritenbaum, C. K. (1984). Household refuse analysis: Basic method and applications to social science. *American Behavioral Scientist, 28,* 5-160.

Reardon, K. K., Sussman, S., & Flay, B. R. (1989). Are we marketing the right message? Can kids really "just say no" to smoking? *Communication Monographs, 56,* 307-324.

Repace, J. L., & Lowrey, A. H. (1987). Predicting the lung cancer risk of domestic passive smoking [Letter]. *American Review of Respiratory Disease, 136*(5), 1308.

Richardson, J. L., Dwyer, K., McGuigan, K., Hansen, W. B., Dent, C., Johnson, C. A., Sussman, S. Y., Brannon, B. R., & Flay, B. R. (1989). Substance use among eighth-grade students who take care of themselves after school. *Pediatrics, 84*(3), 556-566.

Rogers, E. M. (1983). *Diffusion of innovations* (3rd ed.). New York: Free Press.

Rogers, R. G., & Crank, J. (1988). Ethnic differences in smoking patterns: Findings from NHIS. *Public Health Reports, 103*(4), 387-393.

Rohrbach, L. A., Graham, J. W., & Hansen, W. B. (1993). Diffusion of a school-based substance abuse prevention program: Predictors of program implementation. *Preventive Medicine, 22,* 237-260.

Rohrbach, L. A., Graham, J. W., Hansen, W. B., Flay, B. R., & Johnson, C. A. (1987). Evaluation of resistance skills training using multitrait-multimethod role play skill assessments. *Health Education Research: Theory and Practice, 2*(4), 401-407.

Rokeach, M. (1973). *The nature of human values.* New York: Free Press.

Rosenberg, M. (1972). *Society and the adolescent self-image.* Princeton, NJ: Princeton University Press.

Rossi, J. S. (1990). Statistical power of psychological research: What have we gained in 20 years? *Journal of Consulting and Clinical Psychology, 58,* 646-656.

Rouse, B. A. (1989). Epidemiology of smokeless tobacco use: A national study. *National Cancer Institute Monographs, 8,* 29-33.

Runkel, P. J., & McGrath, J. E. (1972). *Research on human behavior: A systematic guide to method.* New York: Holt, Rinehart & Winston.

Russell, M.A.H. (1986). Smoking as a dependence disorder. In L. M. Ramstrom (Ed.), *The smoking epidemic, a matter of worldwide concern.* Stockholm: Almqvist & Wiskell International.

Sackett, G. P. (Ed.). (1978). *Observing behavior: Vol. 2. Data collection and analysis methods.* Baltimore: University Park Press.

Salomon, G., Stein, Y., Eisenberg, S., & Klein, L. (1984). Adolescent smokers and nonsmokers: Profiles and their changing structure. *Preventive Medicine, 13,* 446-461.

Sarvela, P. D., & McClendon, E. J. (1987). An impact evaluation of a rural youth drug education program. *Journal of Drug Education, 17*(3), 213-231.

Schinke, S. P., & Gilchrist, L. D. (1985). Preventing substance abuse with children and adolescents. *Journal of Consulting and Clinical Psychology, 53,* 596-602.

Schinke, S. P., Gilchrist, L. D., Schilling, R. F., Snow, W. H., & Bobo, J. K. (1986). Skills training to prevent smoking. *Health Education Quarterly, 13,* 23-27.

Schmidt, F. (1986). Are there allergic reactions to tobacco smoke? One overview. *Allergologies, 9*(10), 435-438.

Schwartz, S. H., & Inbar-Saban, N. (1988). Value self-confrontation as a method to aid in weight loss. *Journal of Personality and Social Psychology, 54,* 396-404.

Selski, E., Craig, S., Barovich, M., & Sussman, S. (1989). *Project Towards No Tobacco Use (TNT): Tobacco use prevention guide, combined curriculum.* Los Angeles: University of Southern California, Institute for Health Promotion and Disease Prevention Research.

Semmer, N. K., Cleary, P. D., Dwyer, J. H., Fuchs, R., & Lippert, P. (1987). Psychosocial predictors of adolescent smoking in two German cities: The Berlin-Breman study. *Morbidity and Mortality Weekly Report Supplement, 36*(45), 3-10.

Severson, H. H. (1992). Enough snuff: Cessation from the behavioral, clinical, and public health perspectives. In R. C. Stotts, K. L. Schroeder, & D. M. Burns (Eds.), *Smokeless tobacco and health: An international perspective. Monograph 2* (DHHS Publication No. 92-3461) (chap. 6). Rockville, MD: U.S. Department of Health and Human Services, National Cancer Institute, Public Health Service.

Severson, H. H., & Ary, D. V. (1983). Sampling bias due to consent procedures with adolescents. *Addictive Behaviors, 8,* 433-437.

Severson, H. H., Glasgow, R., Wirt, R., Zoref, L., Black, C., Biglan, A., Ary, D., Ochs, L., Weissman, W., & Brozovsky, P. (1991). Preventing the use of smokeless tobacco and cigarettes by teens: Results of a classroom intervention. *Health Education Research: Theory and Practice, 6*(1), 109-120.

Shapiro, A. K., & Morris, L. A. (1971). The placebo effect in medical and psychological therapies. In A. E. Bergin & S. L. Garfield (Eds.), *Handbook of psychotherapy and behavior change* (pp. 369-410, 437-473). New York: John Wiley.

Shiffman, S. (1982). Relapse following smoking cessation: A situational analysis. *Journal of Consulting and Clinical Psychology, 50,* 71-86.

Shiffman, S. (1984). Coping with temptations to smoke. *Journal of Consulting and Clinical Psychology, 52,* 261-267.

Shiffman, S. (1986). A cluster-analytic classification of smoking relapse episodes. *Addictive Behaviors, 11,* 295-307.

Shrum, W., & Cheek, N. H. (1987). Social structure during the school years: Onset of the degrouping process. *American Sociological Review, 52,* 218-223.

Silvestri, B., & Flay, B. R. (1989). Smoking education: Comparison of practice and state-of-the-art. *Preventive Medicine, 18,* 257-266.

Simon, T. R., Sussman, S., Dent, C. W., Burton, D., & Flay, B. R. (1993). Correlates of exclusive or combined use of cigarettes and smokeless tobacco among male adolescents. *Addictive Behaviors, 18,* 623-634.

Skager, R., & Fisher, D. G. (1994). *Substance use among high school students in relation to school characteristics.* Manuscript submitted for publication.

Skinner, W. B., Massey, J. L., Krohn, M. D., & Lauer, R. M. (1985). Social influences and constraints on the initiation and cessation of adolescent tobacco use. *Journal of Behavioral Medicine, 8,* 353-376.

Sobel, M. E. (1982). Asymptotic confidence intervals for indirect effects in structural equation models. In S. Leinhard (Ed.), *Sociological methodology 1982* (pp. 290-293). Washington, DC: American Sociological Association.

Sobol, D. F., Rohrbach, L. A., Dent, C. W., Gleason, L., Brannon, B. R., Johnson, C. A., & Flay, B. R. (1989). The integrity of smoking prevention curriculum delivery. *Health Education Research: Theory and Practice, 4,* 59-67.

Stacy, A. W. (1994). *Memory association in models of alcohol and marijuana use.* Manuscript submitted for publication.

Stacy, A. W., Dent, C. W., Sussman, S., Raynor, A., Burton, D., & Flay, B. R. (1990). Expectancy accessibility and the influence of outcome expectancies on adolescent smokeless tobacco use. *Journal of Applied Social Psychology, 20*(10), 802-817.

Stacy, A. W., Flay, B. R., Sussman, S., Brown, K. S., Santi, S., & Best, J. A. (1990). Validity of alternative self-report indices of smoking among adolescents. *Psychological Assessment: A Journal of Consulting and Clinical Psychology, 2,* 442-446.

Stacy, A. W., Galaif, E. R., Sussman, S., & Dent, C. W. (1994). *Perceived drug outcomes in high risk Latino and non-Hispanic white adolescents.* Manuscript submitted for publication.

Stacy, A. W., Leigh, B. C., & Weingardt, K. (in press). Memory accessibility and association of alcohol use and its positive outcomes. *Experimental and Clinical Psychopharmacology.*

Stacy, A. W., MacKinnon, D. P., & Pentz, M. A. (1993). Generality and specificity in health behavior: Application to warning-label and social influence expectancies. *Journal of Applied Psychology, 78*(4), 611-627.

Stacy, A. W., Sussman, S., Dent, C. W., Burton, D., & Flay, B. R. (1992). Moderators of social influence in adolescent smoking. *Personality and Social Psychology Bulletin, 18*(2), 163-172.

Stacy, A. W., Sussman, S., Hansen, W. B., Johnson, C. A, & Flay, B. R. (1993). *Social influence variables as predictors of later cigarette smoking.* Unpublished manuscript.

Stacy, A. W., Widaman, K. F., & Marlatt, G. A. (1990). Expectancy models of alcohol use. *Journal of Personality and Social Psychology, 58,* 918-928.

Stern, R. A., Prochaska, J. R., Velicer, W. F., & Elder, J. P. (1987). Stages of adolescent cigarette smoking acquisition: Measurement and sample profiles. *Addictive Behaviors, 12,* 319-329.

Stevens, V. J., Severson, H., Lichtenstein, E., Little, S. J., & Leben, J. (1992, May). *Making the most of a teachable moment: smokeless tobacco intervention in the dental office setting.* Paper presented at the Expert Advisory Group on the Essential Elements of Spitting Tobacco Prevention and Cessation Programs, National Cancer Institute, Rockville, MD.

Stewart, D. W., & Shamdasani, P. M. (1990). *Focus groups: Theory and practice.* Newbury Park, CA: Sage.

Sussman, S. (1987). *Smokeless tobacco: Onset, prevention and cessation.* Unpublished grant proposal to the National Cancer Institute.

Sussman, S. (1989). Two social influence perspectives of tobacco use development and prevention. *Health Education Research: Theory and Practice, 4,* 213-223.

Sussman, S. (1991). Curriculum development in school-based prevention research. *Health Education Research: Theory and Practice, 6,* 339-351.

Sussman, S., Brannon, B. R., Dent, C. W., Hansen, W. B., Johnson, C. A., & Flay, B. R. (1993). Relations of coping effort, coping strategies, perceived stress, and cigarette smoking among adolescents. *International Journal of the Addictions, 28*(7), 599-612.

Sussman, S., Brannon, B. R., Flay, B. R., Gleason, L., Senor, S., Sobol, D. F., Hansen, W. B., & Johnson, C. A. (1986). The television, school, and family smoking prevention/cessation project: II. Formative evaluation of televised segments by teenagers and parents—Implications for parental involvement in drug education. *Health Education Research: Theory and Practice, 1*, 185-194.

Sussman, S., Burton, D., Dent, C. W., Stacy, A., & Flay, B. R. (1991). Use of focus groups in developing an adolescent tobacco use prevention program: Collective norm effects. *Journal of Applied Social Psychology, 21*, 1772-1782.

Sussman, S., Dent, C. W., Brannon, B. R., Glowacz, K., Gleason, L. R., Ullery, S., Hansen, W. B., Johnson, C. A., & Flay, B. R. (1989). The television, school and family smoking prevention/cessation project. IV. Controlling for program success expectancies across experimental and control conditions. *Addictive Behaviors, 14*, 601-610.

Sussman, S., Dent, C. W., Flay, B. R., Burton, D., Craig, S., Mestel-Rauch, J., & Holden, S. (1989). Media manipulation of adolescents' personal level judgments regarding consequences of smokeless tobacco use. *Journal of Drug Education, 19*, 43-57.

Sussman, S., Dent, C. W., Flay, B. R., Hansen, W. B., & Johnson, C. A. (1987). Psychosocial predictors of cigarette smoking onset by white, black, Hispanic and Asian adolescents in Southern California. *Morbidity and Mortality Weekly Report Supplement, 36*, 11-16.

Sussman, S., Dent, C. W., McAdams, L. A., Stacy, A. W., Burton, D., & Flay, B. R. (1994). Peer group association and adolescent tobacco use: A one-year prospective study. *Journal of Abnormal Psychology, 103*, 576-580.

Sussman, S., Dent, C. W., Mestel-Rauch, J. S., Johnson, C. A., Hansen, W. B., & Flay, B. R. (1988). Adolescent nonsmokers, triers, and regular smokers' estimates of cigarette smoking prevalence: When do overestimations occur and by whom? *Journal of Applied Social Psychology, 18*, 537-551.

Sussman, S., Dent, C. W., Raynor, A., Stacy, A., Charlin, V., Craig, S., Hansen, W. B., Burton, D., & Flay, B. R. (1988). *The relevance of peer group association to adolescent tobacco use.* Poster presentation at the Third Behavior Therapy World Congress, September, Edinburgh, UK.

Sussman, S., Dent, C. W., Simon, T. R., Stacy, A. W., Burton, D., & Flay, B. R. (1993). Identification of which high-risk youth smoke cigarettes regularly. *Health Values, 17*(1), 42-53.

Sussman, S., Dent, C. W., Simon, T. R., Stacy, A. W., Galaif, E. R., Moss, M. A., Craig, S., & Johnson, C. A. (in press). Effectiveness of social influence substance abuse prevention curricula in comprehensive and continuation high schools. *Drugs and Society.*

Sussman, S., Dent, C. W., Stacy, A. W., Burciaga, C., Raynor, A., Turner, G. E., Charlin, V., Craig, S., Hansen, W. B., Burton, D., & Flay, B. R. (1990). Peer group association and adolescent tobacco use. *Journal of Abnormal Psychology, 99*,(4) 349-352.

Sussman, S., Dent, C. W., Stacy, A. W., Burton, D., & Flay, B. R. (1989). [Self-reported addiction to tobacco products in southern California and Illinois high schools, Year 2 high school survey of Project Towards No Tobacco Use.] Unpublished data.

Sussman, S., Dent, C. W., Stacy, A. W., Burton, D., & Flay, B. R. (1992). [Recall of placement of "booster posters" in all high school ninth-grade classrooms, Year 5 posttest of Project Towards No Tobacco Use.] Unpublished data.

Sussman, S., Dent, C. W., Stacy, A. W., Burton, D., & Flay, B. R. (in press). Psychosocial predictors of health risk factors in adolescents. *Journal of Pediatric Psychology.*

Sussman, S., Dent, C. W., Stacy, A. W., Burton, D., & Flay, B. R. (1994). Psychosocial variables as prospective predictors of violent events among adolescents. *Health Values, 8*(3), 29-40.

Sussman, S., Dent, C. W., Stacy, A. W., Hodgson, C. S., Burton, D., & Flay, B. R. (1993c). Implementation, process, and immediate outcome evaluation of Project Towards No Tobacco Use. *Health Education Research: Theory and Practice, 8,* 109-123.

Sussman, S., Dent, C. W., Stacy, A. W., Sun, P., Craig, S., Simon, T. R., Burton, D., & Flay, B. R. (1993). Project Towards No Tobacco Use: One-year behavior outcomes. *American Journal of Public Health, 83,* 1245-1250.

Sussman, S., Flay, B. R., Budd, R., Brannon, B. R., Gleason, L. R., Glowacz, K. M., & Dent, C. W. (1986). *Student pretest and posttest questionnaire development and content: Television, school and family project* (Technical Report #86-TVSFP-14). Los Angeles: University of Southern California, Health Behavior Research Institute.

Sussman, S., Flay, B. R., Sobel, J. L., Rauch, J., Hansen, W. B., & Johnson, C. A. (1989). Viewing and evaluation of a televised drug education program by students previously or concurrently exposed to school-based substance abuse prevention programming. *Health Education Research: Theory and Practice, 2,* 373-384.

Sussman, S., Galaif, J., Charlin, V., Dent, C. W., Craig, S., Hahn, G., Klein-Selski, E., Barovich, M., & Abrams, C. (1989). TNT Prevention Development (Technical Report #89-TNT-02). University of Southern California, Institute for Health Promotion and Disease Prevention Research.

Sussman, S., Hahn, G., Dent, C. W., Stacy, A. W., Burton, C., & Flay, B. R. (1993). Naturalistic observation of adolescent tobacco use. *International Journal of the Addictions, 28,* 803-811.

Sussman, S., Simon, T. R., & Stacy, A. W. (1994). *Researchers' use of the term "high risk": A psychINFO scan of the literature.* Manuscript submitted for publication.

Sussman, S., Stacy, A. W., Dent, C. W., Burciaga, C., Burton, D., & Flay, B. R. (1993). Refusal assertion versus conversational skill role-play competence: Relevance to prediction of tobacco use. *Statistics in Medicine, 12*(3/4), 365-376.

Sussman, S., Stacy, A. W., Dent, C. W., Simon, T. R., Galaif, E. R., Moss, M. A., Craig, S., & Johnson, C. A. (in press). Continuation high schools: Youth at risk for drug abuse. *Journal of Drug Education.*

Sussman, S., Whitney-Saltiel, D., Budd, R. J., Spiegel, D., Brannon, B. R., Hansen, W. B., Johnson, C. A., & Flay, B. R. (1989). Joiners and non-joiners in worksite smoking treatment: Pretreatment smoking, smoking by significant others, and expectation to quit as predictors. *Addictive Behaviors, 14*(2), 113-119.

Sutton, S. R., & Eiser, J. R. (1984). The effect of fear-arousing communications on cigarette smoking: An expectancy-value approach. *Journal of Behavioral Medicine, 7*(1), 13-33.

Swan, N. (1993). Despite advances, drug craving remains an elusive research target. *NIDA Notes, 8*(2), 1, 4-5.

Swisher, J. D., & Hu, T.-W. (1983). Alternatives to drug abuse: Some are and some are not. In T. J. Glynn, C. G. Leukefeld, & J. P. Ludford (Eds.), *Preventing adolescent drug abuse: Intervention strategies* (NIDA Research Monograph 47) (pp. 141-153). Rockville, MD: National Institute on Drug Abuse.

Thompson, E. L. (1978). Smoking education programs, 1960-1976. *American Journal of Public Health, 68,* 250-257.

Tobler, N. S. (1986). Meta-analysis of 143 adolescent drug prevention programs: Quantitative outcomes results of program participants compared to a control or comparison group. *Journal of Drug Issues, 16,* 535-567.

Tomkins, S. S. (1966). Psychological model for smoking behavior. *American Journal of Public Health, 56,* 17-20.

Tow, P. K., & Smith, P. N. (1988). Writing activities in the health education classroom. *Journal of School Health, 58,* 29-31.

Tricker, R., & Davis, L. G. (1988). Implementing drug education in schools: An analysis of the costs and teacher perceptions. *Journal of School Health, 58,* 181-185.

Turner, G. E., Burciaga, C., Sussman, S., Klein-Selski, E., Craig, S., Dent, C. W., Mason, H., Burton, D., & Flay, B. R. (1993). Which lesson components mediate refusal assertion skill improvement in school-based adolescent tobacco use prevention? *International Journal of the Addictions, 28*(8), 749-766.

Tyler, T. R., & Cook, F. L. (1984). The mass media and judgements of risk: Distinguishing impact on personal and societal level judgments. *Journal of Personality and Social Psychology, 47,* 693-708.

Upshaw, H. S., & Ostrom, T. M. (1984). Psychological perspective in attitude research. In J. R. Eiser (Ed.), *Attitudinal judgment* (pp. 23-42). New York: Springer-Verlag.

Urberg, K. A., Cheng, C., & Shyu, S. (1991). Grade changes in peer influence on adolescent cigarette smoking: A comparison of two measures. *Addictive Behaviors, 16,* 21-28.

U.S. Bureau of the Census. (1983, April). *1980 Census of Population and Housing: Geographic identification code scheme* (Census publication PHC80-R5). Washington, DC: Author.

U.S. Department of Health and Human Services (U.S. DHHS). (1984). *The health consequences of smoking: Chronic obstructive lung disease. A report of the Surgeon General* (Publication No. DHHS [PHS] 84-50205). Washington, DC: Public Health Service, Office on Smoking and Health.

U.S. Department of Health and Human Services (U.S. DHHS). (1985). *The health consequences of smoking: Cancer and chronic lung disease in the workplace. A report of the Surgeon General* (DHHS Publication No. [PHS] 85-50207. Washington, DC: Public Health Service, Office on Smoking and Health.

U.S. Department of Health and Human Services (U.S. DHHS). (1986). *The health consequences of using smokeless tobacco: A report of the Advisory Committee to the Surgeon General* (Publication No. NIH 85-2874). Washington, DC: Public Health Service.

U.S. Department of Health and Human Services (U.S. DHHS). (1988). *The health consequences of smoking: Nicotine addiction. A report of the Surgeon General, 1988* (DHHS Publication No. [CDC] 88-8406). Washington, DC: Public Health Service, Centers for Disease Control, Center for Chronic Disease Prevention and Health Promotion, Office on Smoking and Health.

U.S. Department of Health and Human Services (U.S. DHHS). (1989). *Reducing the health consequences of smoking: 25 years of progress. A report of the Surgeon General* (DHHS Publication No. [CDC] 89-8411). Washington, DC: Public Health Service.

U.S. Department of Health and Human Services (U.S. DHHS). (1990). *Smoking, Tobacco, and Cancer Program: 1985-1989 status report* (NIH Publication No. 90-3107). Washington, DC: National Institutes of Health.

U.S. Department of Health and Human Services (U.S. DHHS). (1991a). *Healthy people 2000: National health promotion and disease prevention objectives, full report, with commentary* (DHHS Publication No. (PHS) 91-50212). Washington, DC: Public Health Service.

U.S. Department of Health and Human Services (U.S. DHHS). (1991b). *Strategies to control tobacco use in the United States: A blueprint for public health action in the 1990's* (Smoking and Tobacco Control Monographs 1, NIH Publication No. 92-3316). Washington, DC: Public Health Service, National Institutes of Health, National Cancer Institute.

U.S. Department of Health and Human Services (U.S. DHHS). (1993). *Respiratory health effects of passive smoking: Lung cancer and other disorders* (NIH Publication No. 93-3605). Washington, DC: U.S. Environmental Protection Agency.

U.S. Department of Health and Human Services (U.S. DHHS). (1994). *Preventing tobacco use among young people: A report of the Surgeon General* (Publication No. S/N 017-001-00491-0). Washington, DC: Public Health Service.

Vartiainen, E., Pallonen, U., McAlister, A., & Puska, P. (1990). Eight-year follow-up results of an adolescent smoking prevention program: The North Karelia project. *American Journal of Public Health, 80,* 78-79.

Velicer, W. F., Prochaska, J. O., Rossi, J. S., & Snow, M. G. (1992). Assessing outcome in smoking cessation studies. *Psychological Bulletin, 111,* 23-41.

Vogt, T. M., Selvin, S., Widdowson, G., & Hulley, S. B. (1977). Expired air carbon monoxide and serum thiocyanate as objective measures of cigarette exposure. *American Journal of Public Health, 67,* 545-549.

Vriend, T. (1969). High-performing inner-city adolescents assist low-performing peers in counseling groups. *Personnel Guidance, 48,* 897-904.

Wallack, L. (1984). Practical issues, ethical concerns and future directions in the prevention of alcohol-related problems. *Journal of Primary Prevention, 4,* 199-224.

Webb, E. J., Campbell, D. T., Schwartz, R. D., & Sechrest, L. (1966). *Unobtrusive measures: Nonreactive research in the social sciences.* Chicago: Rand McNally.

Weinstein, N. D. (1982). Unrealistic optimism about susceptibility to health problems. *Journal of Behavioral Medicine, 5,* 441-460.

Williams, C. L., Eng, A., Botvin, G. J., Hill, P. H., & Ernst, L. W. (1979). Validation of students self-reported cigarette smoking status with plasma cotinine levels. *American Journal of Public Health, 69*(12), 1272-1274.

Wills, T. A. (1985). Supportive functions of interpersonal relationships. In S. Cohen & S. L. Symes (Eds.), *Social support and health* (pp. 23-42). New York: Academic Press.

Wills, T. A. (1986). Stress and coping in early adolescence: Relationships to substance use in urban school samples. *Health Psychology, 5,* 503-529.

Wills, T. A., Baker, E., & Botvin, G. J. (1989). Dimensions of assertiveness: Differential relationships to substance use in early adolescence. *Journal of Consulting and Clinical Psychology, 57,* 473-478.

Wimmer, R. D., & Dominick, J. R. (1987). *Mass media research.* Belmont, CA: Wadsworth.

Worden, J. K., Flynn, B. S., Geller, B. M., Chen, M., Shelton, L. G., Secker-Walker, R. H., Solomon, D. S., Solomon, L. J., Couchey, S., & Costanza, M. C. (1988). Development of a smoking prevention mass media program using diagnostic and formative research. *Preventive Medicine, 17,* 531-558.

Wydner, E., & Hoffman, D. (1979). Tobacco and health—Societal challenge. *New England Journal of Medicine, 300,* 894-903.

Wyer, R. S., & Srull, T. K. (1989). *Memory and cognition in its social context.* Hillsdale, NJ: Lawrence Erlbaum.

Yalom, I. D. (1975). *The theory and practice of group psychotherapy.* New York: Basic Books.

Young, R. L., Elder, J. P., Green, M., de Moor, C., & Wildey, M. B. (1988). Tobacco use prevention and health facilitator effectiveness. *Journal of School Health, 58,* 370-373.

Zavela, K. J., Harrison, L. R., & Owens, S. (1991, November). *Factors related to smokeless tobacco cessation in young adults.* Poster presentation at American Public Health Association 119th Annual Meeting, Alcohol, Tobacco and Other Drugs Section, Atlanta.

Index

About the Authors

Steve Sussman, Ph.D., received his doctorate in clinical-social psychology from the University of Illinois at Chicago in 1984. He served on a clinical psychology residency at Jackson Veterans Administration and University of Mississippi Medical Centers and now is an Associate Professor of Preventive Medicine at the University of Southern California. He has published over 60 articles in the area of drug use prevention and cessation. Subareas of particular focus are psychosocial prediction of tobacco and other drug use, school-based tobacco and other drug use prevention and cessation, and relapse prevention.

Clyde W. Dent, Ph.D., received his doctorate in quantitative psychology from the Psychology Department at the University of North Carolina, Chapel Hill, in 1984. He is an Associate Professor of Research at the University of Southern California. His current areas of interest include methodological and applied issues in biometrics, quantitative psychology, and behavioral statistics.

Alan W. Stacy, Ph.D., received his doctorate in social/personality psychology from the University of California, Riverside, in 1986. He is currently a Research Associate Professor of Preventive Medicine at USC. His primary research interests are in development of memory models of health behavior, as applied to etiology, prevention, and treatment. Also, he has interests in theories of expectancy processes and social influence.

Dee Burton, Ph.D., received her doctorate in social/personality psychology from The New School for Social Research, New York, in 1977. She has a current research focus in adolescent tobacco use cessation, confirmed smokers, and ethnic and cultural differences in use of mass media and response to advertising. Her published research includes articles on heavy smokers, smoking imagery among youth, locus of control factors in smoking, and cross-cultural differences in use of the mass media. She is the Associate Director of Media Research of the University of Illinois at the Chicago Prevention Research Center and Associate Professor in the School of Public Health.

Brian R. Flay, Ph.D., received his doctorate in social psychology from Waikato University in New Zealand in 1976. After receiving postdoctoral training at Northwestern University (Evanston, Illinois) under a Fullbright/Hays Fellowship, he started research on smoking prevention at the University of Waterloo (Ontario, Canada). He continued work on smoking prevention and developed work in the areas of drug use prevention and the use of mass media for smoking cessation at the University of Southern California. He is currently Director of the Prevention Research Center and Associate Professor in the School of Public Health at the University of Illinois at Chicago, where he continues his research in the above areas, as well as the areas of AIDS and violence prevention.

C. Anderson Johnson, Ph.D., received his doctorate in Social Psychology from Duke University in 1974. He was Assistant Professor at the University of Minnesota from 1975 to 1980. Since 1980 he has been Associate Professor of Preventive Medicine at the University of Southern California and Director of the USC Institute for Health Promotion and Disease Prevention Research. He has received support from the National Cancer Institute, the National Heart, Lung, and Blood Institute, the National Institute for Child Health and Human Development, the National Institute on Drug Abuse, the W.T. Grant Foundation, and the Kaiser Family Foundation. He is currently Sidney R. Garfield Chair in Health Sciences at the University of Southern California.